THE CHALLENGES OF WORKING WITH CHILD SEXUAL EXPLOITATION AND HOW A PSYCHOANALYTIC UNDERSTANDING CAN HELP

Sexual exploitation is becoming endemic in our society. It involves victims being coerced to enter abusive sexual relationships with individuals or gangs. It can occur with children from care homes – or from more privileged backgrounds. Sexual exploitation is so addictive that it is really difficult to extract the victims. This is the first book that we are aware of that examines exploitation using a psychoanalytic framework which makes the behaviour and motives of victims and, in some cases, exploiters comprehensible. The book looks at a range of situations from care homes to refugee camps and elite schools.

We expect this book to become indispensable for social workers, psychotherapists, counsellors, and care workers who have to tackle child sexual exploitation. Giving up an addiction is a struggle. Our clinical examples show how much and what kinds of work are needed to start to release girls from their addiction to their exploiters.

The roots of vulnerability lie in an attack on the maternal function. This is reflected in the huge expansion of day-care taking children from as little as three months old. Care for mothers and children can be transformed. We demonstrate how powerful properly organised maternal-type care can be, to give young people a sound start to their lives.

Marion Bower has postgraduate diplomas in Education and Social Work. She was a Consultant Social Worker at the Tavistock Clinic and is a Senior Adult Psychotherapist. She has written and edited four books on related subjects and is currently working on a biography of Psychoanalyst Melanie Klein, to be published by Routledge.

Robin Solomon has been a Clinical Social Worker/Psychotherapist for over 40 years. She has held senior posts at the Tavistock Clinic as a clinician and as an educator. She now works independently as an external staff consultant with CAMHS services in Britain and abroad and with residential care homes for Looked After adolescents.

THE CHALLENGES OF WORKING WITH CHILD SEXUAL EXPLOITATION AND HOW A PSYCHOANALYTIC UNDERSTANDING CAN HELP

Edited by Marion Bower and Robin Solomon

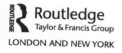

Routledge
Taylor & Francis Group

LONDON AND NEW YORK

Designed cover image: © Maggie Garson 2023

First published 2024
by Routledge
4 Park Square, Milton Park, Abingdon, Oxon OX14 4RN

and by Routledge
605 Third Avenue, New York, NY 10158

Routledge is an imprint of the Taylor & Francis Group, an informa business

© 2024 selection and editorial matter, Marion Bower and Robin Solomon; individual chapters, the contributors

British Library Cataloguing-in-Publication Data
A catalogue record for this book is available from the British Library

Library of Congress Cataloging-in-Publication Data
Names: Bower, Marion, 1949- editor. | Solomon, Robin (Social worker), editor.
Title: The challenges of working with child sexual exploitation and how a psychoanalytic understanding can help / edited by Marion Bower and Robin Solomon.
Description: Abingdon, Oxon ; New York, NY : Routledge, 2024. | Includes bibliographical references and index. |
Identifiers: LCCN 2023056466 (print) | LCCN 2023056467 (ebook) | ISBN 9780367896645 (hardback) | ISBN 9780367896638 (paperback) | ISBN 9781003020370 (ebook)
Subjects: LCSH: Sexually abused children--Rehabilitation. | Sexually abused children--Mental health services. | Sexually abused children--Psychology. | Child sexual abuse--Psychological aspects. | Child analysis.
Classification: LCC RJ507.S49 C43 2024 (print) | LCC RJ507.S49 (ebook) | DDC 362.76--dc23/eng/20240221
LC record available at https://lccn.loc.gov/2023056466
LC ebook record available at https://lccn.loc.gov/2023056467

ISBN: 978-0-367-89664-5 (hbk)
ISBN: 978-0-367-89663-8 (pbk)
ISBN: 978-1-003-02037-0 (ebk)

DOI: 10.4324/9781003020370

Typeset in Sabon
by KnowledgeWorks Global Ltd.

CONTENTS

CONTRIBUTORS

Steve Bambrough is the Associate Director of Clinical Services at the Tavistock & Portman NHS Foundation Trust. Steve is a registered social worker with Social Work England. He qualified as a social worker in 1995 and worked as a social worker in local authority and charitable sector before joining the Tavistock Clinic in 2003.

Marion Bower has postgraduate diplomas in Education and Social Work. She was a Consultant Social Worker at the Tavistock Clinic and is a Senior Adult Psychotherapist. She has written and edited four books on related subjects and is currently working on a biography of Psychoanalyst Melanie Klein to be published by Routledge.

Krisna Catsaras is a Child and Adolescent Psychotherapist with a particular interest in intercultural and transnational work. He works in the National Health Service (NHS) and private practice. Krisna also offers organisational and leadership consultancy, usually to public and third sector organisations working with children and young people.

Janine Cherry-Swaine is a consultant psychotherapist in the NHS. She trained at the Tavistock Clinic as a child and adolescent psychotherapist and later as an organisational consultant. She consults to a variety of services and organisations on workplace post incident response and on the impact of vicarious sexual trauma upon team and organisational effectiveness.

Fiona Henderson is a Clinical Psychologist and Psychoanalytic Psychotherapist who has worked in adult and family mental health services. She was a consultant adult psychotherapist at the Tavistock Clinic. She has published papers on psychotherapy with mothers who have harmed their children and on the dynamics of difficult conversations in social work.

Julie Long is a Tavistock Clinic trained Consultant Child and Adolescent Psychotherapist. She worked for Westminster Social Services and with highly traumatised adolescents at the Cassel Hospital. She is an ACP Training analyst and an Adult and Child Psychoanalyst with the British Psychoanalytic Association (BPA). She currently works in private practise in West London.

Ariel Nathanson is a Consultant Child, Adolescent and Adult Psychotherapist. He is the under 21's clinical lead at the Portman Clinic and consults to other care organisations. He specialises in work with young people who display sexually harmful, delinquent, and violent behaviours and has co-edited work on this subject.

Alison Roy is a Consultant Child Psychotherapist and Psychotherapist. She worked in the NHS for over 25 years and is now in independent practice. She was the co-founder and Clinical Lead for AdCAMHS, a specialist adoption service. She has written *A For Adoption* (2020) and a chapter in *Education through the Art* (2021).

R.M. Shingleton is a Local Authority Children's Service Social Worker and was previously an Integrative Therapist in schools and the charitable sector.

Robin Solomon has been a Clinical Social Worker/Psychotherapist for over 40 years. She has held senior posts at the Tavistock Clinic as a clinician and as an educator. She now works independently as an external staff consultant with CAMHS services in Britain and abroad and with residential care homes for Looked After adolescents.

Judith Trowell is a Consultant Child and Adolescent Psychiatrist, an Adult Psychoanalyst, a Child Analyst, and a Founder of Young Minds. She was the Tavistock Clinic Head of the Department of Children and Parents, professor of Child Mental Health in the West Midlands and at Worcester University, and has led clinical outcome research studies.

ACKNOWLEDGEMENTS

We are very grateful to all our contributors who have worked hard to present clear accounts of immensely demanding work.

Robin and Marion would also like to thank Steve Bower without whom this book would not exist. Many thanks to Maggie Garson for the powerful image we use on the front cover of this book.

Thanks also to Claire Jarvis and Sully Evans, our editors at Routledge, for their support and patience.

1

INTRODUCTION

This book reflects the challenges that everyone faces when they try to work with young people caught up in being sexually exploited or moving on after exploitation. All our case material is anonymised but shows the huge difficulties that vulnerable and sexually exploited young people have faced and still face in moving on. The key to our understanding has been the extent that missing maternal care as a newly born child and in early years can make young people catastrophically vulnerable. Older children, adults or gangs exploit what their target children have missed and can groom them to accept perverse sexual relationships as part of a package that appears to offer the care that they have never had.

The first chapters in the book present specific cases and specific examples of how difficult it is to make meaningful contact and progress meaningful work with exploited young people in individual therapy. We broaden the view to show the difficulties of responses of multiple organisations. The government is aware of reports examining the failures of multiple agencies, specifically in Rotherham. We have a first-hand view of the first pilot agency set up in Rotherham to respond to damning criticisms of the Rotherham failures picked up by reports of Inquiry by Baroness Jay.

The second half of the book broadens our view. Chapters review the social and political context and experience in research where exploitation was suspected but denied over many years. Experienced practitioners reflect on how consultation can provide essential support to front line workers both in Britain and with refugee children.

Each contribution reflects how difficult it is for exploited young people to engage with any help. Our contributions make clear how limited the changes are for clients following even the most intensive therapy and sheltered settings.

DOI: 10.4324/9781003020370-1

Finally, we consider the damage caused by inadequate care in the early years. There are some cost-effective changes that could be made. Wider partnerships between social workers and other specialists could help. Social worker training could usefully include psychoanalytic views that would radically improve workers' understanding of their clients. All these changes, however, challenge a prevailing British culture that ignores the importance of mothers and maternal care.

We hope that this book will contribute to understanding and advance better approaches to a group of very emotionally damaged young people. People will find what interests them most in different chapters. It will at least help those involved to recognise how difficult this work is. Even best practise can only make very limited improvements to the young people affected. Major social changes are needed. The care safety net must provide maternal-style care for young people. Only this could begin to reduce their vulnerability and improve their lives.

2

EXCITEMENT AS A DEFENCE AGAINST DESPAIR

An adolescent girl's failed mourning of childhood and childhood attachments

Julie Long

> It is my world, not yours ... mine. If you take it away, I will have nothing. There is nothing worse than nothing.
>
> (Jemma, 16 years old)[1]

This chapter explores some of the very real challenges which arise when working, therapeutically, with a particular group of adolescent girls who have experienced sexual exploitation by the hands of predatory paedophile groups. These girls can be rigidly secretive, suspicious and hard to make contact with. States of mind can oscillate between moments of object relating, which supports development (i.e., the child wanting/asking for help), to then, defensively, turning against any awareness of dependency or needing others by turning towards more narcissistic destructive states of mind. In these moments it can feel as though the girls move into an excited identification with those who they feel capture them and abuse them. What makes the work so difficult is the degree to which the sexually violent and perverse nature of the world they have endured, within the paedophile ring, can take on a compelling and addictive quality to it.

These girls have often been groomed, mainly by men outside of the family, where they have been gradually coerced and then forced into sexual activity with multiple men, being passed through a network of perpetrators, across and between towns.

The extreme vulnerability around challenging the narcissistic structure makes therapeutic intervention precarious. Unconsciously, there is often a terror that turning towards a caring object who has the potential to understand the girl's internal predicament (i.e., her longing to be contained and

DOI: 10.4324/9781003020370-2

loved) can lead to a psychic collapse into states of despair. These states are characterised by a severe loss of sense of self, self-hatred and an increased risk of self-harm and suicidality.

Furthermore, it is a core issue for those attempting to care for them or to provide therapy. The experience of 'care' can lead to the girl's awareness of her own vulnerability/dependency needs, which can then lead to flights from treatment and premature endings. The girls I have worked with have all experienced significant loss and trauma that predates the world of sexual exploitation. They have lost their early emotional containment in relationship with their primary maternal figure. This primary failure of early emotional containment in early childhood is a major factor in the girl's vulnerability for sexual exploitation.

This chapter aims to explore the underlying dynamics which emerged in the work with Jemma, who, from the age of 15 years old, was in psychoanalytic treatment which lasted for 3 years. By illustrating the powerful dynamics in the therapeutic relationship and the overwhelming demands placed upon the clinician and the professionals around her, I hope to bring further understanding of how trauma in the earliest relationship resurfaces in adolescence and provides a unique opportunity for new understanding and ways of relating.

The clinical example aims to illustrate the precarious nature of Jemma's internal world. It is dominated by paranoid and hostile relations in which she feels herself to be inhabited and trapped, predominantly by female figures who are either felt to be intrusive, controlling and rivalrous or by passive onlookers to the abuse taking place and impotent to help. The way in which this manifests itself in the analytic work is through the transference and countertransference relationship, one in which the pervasive use of splitting and projective identification aim to defensively freeze the life and any authentic development within the therapeutic relationship and within herself.

My thought is not only of these girls' unexpressed hostility and rivalry with their mother, which is feared, but also that of the internal mother's hostile rivalrous internal objects, all of which are felt to be deeply lodged within her. She fears that these internal objects prevent her from being able to feel that her own needs/hostile or libidinal impulses could be tolerated and contained. Therefore, any attempt she makes to form and develop a relationship, with those trying to care for her, though longed for, is felt to be dangerous and frightening. In defence against any awareness of vulnerability, the adolescent girl can omnipotently take flight by identifying with the sexualised adult world of the parental figures, joining them instead of mourning the loss of her attachments to them.

In this chapter, I will first, briefly, consider the ordinary developmental tasks of adolescence in particular. These are the adolescent's capacity to mourn the loss of earlier childhood attachments from parental figures, to tolerate separateness and turn towards peer relations and authentic adolescent psycho-sexual development. I will then describe the impact that trauma and neglect in the early mother-infant relationship can lead to disturbances at puberty and during adolescence. Deprivation and trauma can impinge and severely inhibit the child's capacity to mourn the attachments of childhood. Instead of working through the pain of detaching their dependency needs from their parents to a peer group, they often feel the compelling 'drive' to 'act' as a means to manage the unbearable pain of separateness.

Adolescence

Adolescence is a developmental process, a period of irreversible physical and emotional changes beginning at puberty. With the loss of childhood and the gradual detachment from parental figures and a change in relationship to authority figures and society, the young person faces intense depressive anxieties.

Bronstein (2020) suggests that during this period, there can be constructive and developmental forces in play in which the young person acquires a new sense of themselves and their physical, mental and emotional capacity. There can be an opening awareness of the body, a new sense of personal experiences. Impulses, powerful inner feelings, thoughts and an increased capacity for reflection can take over in a concrete and compulsive way. Ambivalent feelings of love and hate, normal and acceptable in childhood, take on a different meaning now, in a sexual and more powerfully strong body.

The reworking of the Oedipus complex heightens when aspects of infantile sexuality reappear. Anxieties linked to guilt regarding their awareness of both sexual and aggressive desires and feelings surface. The need to detach themselves from family as love objects and the accompanying oedipal anxieties and to look outwards to others outside the family is essential. Adolescents ordinarily turn towards peer groups who can help contain and manage conflicting feelings. These include further guilt that the new peer group can offer such sanctuary to new thoughts and ideals separate from their parents.

By the end of adolescence, a young person has moved from living in a child's body to living in an adult one, now sexually mature and physically strong. Passivity to the parents has become active with the young person taking responsibility for her own care, feeling more independent and responsible for themselves without being overwhelmed by anxiety. Facing the tasks of ordinary adolescence means bringing together the differing unintegrated infantile sexual aspects of the child under the primacy of the genital and the move to a more mature love and sexual object.

Polmear (2010) suggests that a disturbed or failed adolescent development occurs when the process of mourning the childhood attachments to the parental figures and their ideals is unable to be faced. The adolescent can retreat from the pain of mourning the attachment to the parental figures, to turn towards or into something destructive and narcissistic and to be captured and held in this retreat. Independence becomes a pseudo-independence. The peer group chosen becomes an ideal destructive one, which provides little in the way of support for authentic development.

Bronstein suggests that destructive forces can bring states of confusion, surprise and passion, an upheaval when anxieties can threaten to inundate the ego with life and death drives and with the inevitable clash between progressive and regressive forces. Laufer (1982) suggests that the adolescent can experience the body, during this time of flux, as the 'originator' of all the disturbing feelings stirred up and a carrier of the identification with the often-hated parents. The body (self) can then become the target of hostility. Laufer (1982) suggests that the failure to face the developmental tasks of adolescence and the failure to work through 'mourning' of childhood attachments can lead to adolescent breakdown.

The teenage girls I have worked with have described their early experiences as having little in the way of ordinary emotional containment. Their histories are complex. Experiences of loss, emotional deprivation/trauma, fractured attachments, neglect and abuse permeated their early lives. Their mothers, mainly, have their own history of trauma, violence and/or depression, drug and alcohol abuse.

The girls often feel let down and betrayed by those who ought to have been caring for them. The inevitable losses placed upon them throughout childhood and then from the demands of adolescence, in which difficulties in separation from the parental figures arise, can feel too much and are unable to be faced. Polmear (2010) likens these failures in development to Freud's notion of melancholia in the sense that, rather than give up the loved and hated figures of one's childhood affection, a compromise is found whereby the oedipal or pre-oedipal parents retain their internal position and become incorporated into the young person's adult sexual identity. Freud (1917)

As described by a 19-year-old following a year of inpatient therapy,

> What makes it worse, is that for all I have been through I have never had a 'real' relationship. What no one understands is that I may have had sex with a lot of men, but I have never had a genuine boyfriend. No one has loved me or wanted to care for me. I know it sounds silly but I'm 19 years old and, in a way, I am still, in my mind, a virgin in that way.

Mainly, these girls have little sense of their own identity. They suffer with extremely low self-esteem and self-hatred. They often feel extremely isolated and depressed, let alone being an authentic sexual being. Jemma represents some of the core issues which emerge in the work with such girls.

Jemma

What struck me most when I met 15-year-old Jemma was how her blonde hair was tightly pulled back from her face emphasising the smoothness of her white skin and the still blueness of her eyes. My first thought was that she resembled a porcelain doll looking completely untouched by what one could describe as the messy and damaged aspects of her life. There was no indication of any anxiety in meeting me, but I did sense a fleeting moment of her hypervigilance when her eyes scanned the room and me before she quickly dropped her gaze as though giving me the impression she hadn't noticed anything.

She sat rigidly in the chair and didn't speak. After a while I suggested it may not be easy coming to a new place and meeting me for the first time. She remained rigid and silent, and I was unsure of how she experienced my words or the sound of my voice. I then tentatively wondered aloud as to whether she had allowed herself to come here today. Whilst keeping the frame of her frozen-like portraiture 'intact', her voice cracked, and in a loud brittle high-pitched tone she screamed:

> They made me come here. It's the people on the unit, they think they know what is best. They say I need to talk to someone about what happened back home. But nothing happened. They don't get it, there is nothing to talk about. There isn't a problem, no problem at all. They say it's all stuck in me and it needs to come out. They think it's to do with men, but that is the other girls, not me. That's what they think, they make it up.
>
> They take my phone and check to see who I call. There are locks on the windows and doors. Why do they do this to me, I haven't done anything wrong and yet they treat me as though I have. I have never done anything that they say I have done. They don't listen, no one listens.

The sound of her voice was in complete contrast to how she looked. Her piercing eyes and accusations against the staff in the children's home had a bludgeoning impact on me. For a while I couldn't think, let alone try and understand what she was trying to communicate. It took a while before I stopped listening to the actual words and took note of the underlying communication – mainly that she felt it was others who controlled her, who got her 'deliberately wrong', 'blamed her'. It was 'they' who carried the need for her to come to see me, not her.

I suggested to her that she seemed scared that I will only see an 'all-wrong version of her' made up from others and that she had little belief

I could listen and to get to know her. She winced and momentarily stopped talking. She fleetingly looked at me and whispered, "I miss my mum and my friend back home, particularly my friend I'm closest too". She said that she knew that things in her life had gone wrong and that she wanted to change if given the chance.

In this moment, she indicated how she could move from a highly paranoid and persecuted state of mind to turn to something softer within herself and between us, the potential capacity to take in something meaningful. Possibly, she could link her longing for real emotional contact with a receptive figure, me, her mother or her own best friend.

However, possibly due to a fleeting awareness of the momentary intimate contact felt between us, she then quickly turned away from her more vulnerable needy self and retreated back into a more omnipotent but persecutory world repeatedly letting me know of her grievances, her sense of feeling misunderstood. She spoke or shouted for the rest of the session (and subsequent ones) in such a way that it seemed she was speaking to no one in particular.

In the early months of her therapy, I endured either a complete silence or else her shouting (with no expectation I could hear what she was saying) that they 'had got it wrong', they didn't listen and 'they were unfair'. I heard of her grievances against the staff on the unit, her social worker, the court system and police. All she felt had 'got it wrong' and made up lies against her. She complained about the mistreatment she had experienced from those who, she felt, ought to be caring for her.

I heard of the other girls on the unit's resentments and betrayals: their running away, their sexual exploits or how, despite the helplessness of the staff, to control the girls; the naughty girls were favoured. Any reference to her mother or extended family was idealised and she complained of being 'stolen' away from her parents by the court system.

Any attempt I would make to acknowledge her being upset or to reflect her feeling of unfairness or of being 'let down' would be responded to by screams of 'shut up just shut up, you're not listening, you don't care' and that I was twisting everything of what she said to make her look bad. She hated hearing my voice and often threatened to leave her therapy for good. And yet, if I spoke very little, she complained that she felt she was too much for me and that I hated her. Her moods were volatile and her threats to abandon the work were frequent and alarming.

For what seemed a long time, the work felt fragmented when what was real and what was phantasy led to states of confusion in me. Jemma's contact with me fluctuated as she struggled with two different aspects of herself which rapidly alternated. There was a part of her that froze herself, negating any awareness of any dependency needs and, in doing so, frustrating the efforts of others to help her. The other, more fleeting appearance was infinitely more needy and vulnerable, one which, once opened, was liable to evoke anxiety, confusion and intense pain. It is this pain, linked to the longing of real emotional contact which she so desperately wished for, that quickly needed to be dismissed and denied by her.

On the one hand, I think she was telling me that she had little expectation that 'words' had any meaning or could be used to help her understand her experiences. Words were either shouted over, used for interruption or to be evacuated. On the other hand, I think she conveyed how her use of words and her complaints conveying her feeling of being 'maliciously misunderstood' and mistreated by others had a destructive excited quality to it.

In further sessions, I began to see the degree to which she gained some perverse satisfaction from the underlying pain linked to these abusive and neglectful relationships, not only with others but with herself as well. She often resorted to contempt and dismissiveness towards those who attempt to help her. It seems that a sado-masochistic element of her functioning and relationships was resorted to in which her emotional pain was converted into sexual excitement.

Mainly, what she appeared to convey was felt to be the expression of a very paranoid internal system in which being controlled was at its core. She described the regime at the children's unit as being like prison and the staff watchful warders, warders who preferred the other girls and gave them privileges. In contrast, her social worker represented the overwhelmed passive inactive figure who did nothing for her and continuously let her down.

I often struggled to find my way around the multiple figures that represented disloyalty, bullying and exploitation by the staff and girls on the unit. She depicted a world in which there was no fair-minded figure to turn to. It often felt she existed in a rigid totalitarian, primitive and paranoid state in which there was no world outside of the toxicity, particularly of female relationships. (Relationships with male figures were not referred to for a long time.)

From my notes early in the work I wrote:

I find myself becoming lost 'inside' what can feel like an extremely paranoid scenario finding myself increasingly unable to differentiate who is doing what to whom and what was real and unreal. I feel useless and unable to find a position to think or reflect. I mainly feel insignificant, isolated as though an outside observer, listening in.

In reflection, I can now see how my experience of feeling 'shut out' from the repetitive ruminations in her mind was her means of unconsciously communicating her own infantile experience with a parental figure who is felt to be 'out of reach' and out of touch with her. In these moments, of which there are many, I become a child version of her, feeling helpless and confused. At other moments, such as when I make my presence known to her, I can then become, in her mind, the demanding narcissistic rivalrous figure she most fears. In these moments, she would say, "it's all about you, I wasn't talking about you, but you've made it about you".

She consistently conveyed how she was unable to distinguish to what degree her perceived 'badness' (monstrous phantasies of her intrusively demanding needs permeated with guilt) led her mother to drink or what degree her mother's destructive projections (psychotic in nature) led Jemma to feel herself full of her mother's monstrousness.

Bion (1962) writes that a child whose projections are not accepted is a child exposed to the experience of an impervious or impermeable object. He or she receives back his unprocessed projections in the shape of 'nameless dread', a terror without content or meaning. Instead of introjecting an object that can understand, the infant builds up internally a 'wilfully misunderstanding object' (Bion, 1962, p. 117). The response to such an object may be to try to get through to it by resorting to continued projective identification with increasing force and frequency.

Gianna Williams (1997) describes a reversal of Bion's (1962) container-contained relationship. The process is the opposite of introjecting the organising Alpha function. A child who is still in need of containment is exposed to the experience of being used as a receptacle of massive parental projections. She suggests that parents, who may be traumatised themselves from childhood, may not only not receive the infant's projections but may also feel driven to divest themselves of their own anxiety, psychic pain and ghosts, using their children as a 'receptacle' for their projections. In such cases, there is a risk of the child becoming 'porous to introjecting a disorganising, disrupting agent in the child's internal world' which, Williams terms 'omega function'. In such instance, she suggests the child may resort to developing a 'no entry defence' as seen in anorexic behaviours and including a resistance to taking in the therapists' interpretations or allowing help from others.

From my experience in the countertransference, I believe Jemma remained not only porous to the disturbances of both her parents, who themselves had difficult childhoods but has felt herself to become, prematurely, the container of the infantile aspects of her mother's mind. I think I have experienced this in the work with her when she indicates an acute sensitivity to my capacity to be receptive, or unreceptive, to the changing atmosphere in the analytic relationship between us. I find she both seeks emotional contact whilst taking flight from it. In these moments, she complains of the people who misunderstand her, who were not around for her or who want to control her.

Tustin (1990) suggests that some mothers, due to their own feelings of loneliness and depression, may have reacted towards their babies as if they were parts of their own bodies, filling in the 'black hole' of their own inadequacy, emptiness and loneliness. This, in turn, can leave infants with a particular sensitivity and aversion to their mother's distress or what Britton (1998, p. 58) has referred to as an 'allergy to otherness'.

From the social work reports, I had learned that Jemma's parents both came from disturbed families themselves. They met on an adolescent unit and had a volatile relationship. When her mother was 18 years old, she became pregnant with Jemma. The parents' relationship became more turbulent, but despite this, Jemma's mother went on to have two further children. Father's outbursts were threatening and violent, not only towards her mother but also later to Jemma and her younger brothers. When Gemma was eight, her father left the family to live with another woman and went on relatively successfully to have a new family. However, her mother, unable to manage without father, fell into a deeper depression and began to drink. Despite being able to take better care of her younger brothers, Jemma was neglected and began to miss school. She found solace with a group of similar girls she hung around with, mainly at night, to manage her isolation and loneliness. The older girls in the group were already participating in minor crimes and had been groomed into sexual activities, drugs and alcohol by young and then older men in the community. Jemma increasingly hung around the streets with these girls, truanting and staying out at night. Her mother could no longer manage her.

It was within this context Jemma gradually found herself increasingly becoming immersed in the world of a very cruel and hostile sexual exploitative gang. Despite efforts from the police and social services and a succession of foster carers, she continued to run away and was repeatedly found in the houses of these men. Eventually, under a full care order, she was removed from her home town to semi-secure unit in another part of the country with little contact with family and friends. It was whilst living in the residential unit that she repeatedly asked to see a therapist, and this was arranged.

She never missed a session, was always on time and, despite her protestations that I was useless or made her worse and that she wasn't coming to the next session, she always ended the session with a thank you and see you tomorrow. She complained that she had 'no need' for therapy and that it was only under the duress and control of the staff that she attended. She was afraid of upsetting the adults around her. She feared provoking an anger that would lead to further retaliatory hostile reactions and worse to being rejected and abandoned by being sent to another placement. She powerfully conveyed the underlying message that she could not hear or bear to listen to her own needs.

For a long time, I just sat in my chair and took the brunt of the onslaught. Her fear was palpable, and for months, any wish for meaningful contact was met with suspicion, paranoia and hostility. I learnt to be patient and not to speak too much. Sitting firm in one's own seat holding the therapeutic boundaries was sometimes the most I was able to achieve in sessions for quite some time.

Over time, I began to speak to her as though she were a very little child, using very simple words and short sentences. I would say things like, "you are upset", "you don't like that, and it hurts". Or "it feels as though whatever I say isn't quite right and maybe this is a feeling that you know lots about". I began to realise that any 'you and me' comments provoked a rage.

This seemed to work as over time, she stopped filling up all the space with her shouting. There were moments, though tenuous, when it felt as though there were two people in the room who could tolerate a little of 'taking in something' from each other.

Very gradually, she began to observe her own reactions. In one session, she said, "sometimes, you know, I just need to come in and be angry at all the frustrations in me". and "when you talk, I think you are just going to scream at me to shut up". In these moments, I began to understand how she experienced her own screams as going into me and her fear was that I was just screaming back at her – a hopeless situation with no sense of any thinking going on in her or me.

The initial frozen impenetrable state of mind, so evident at the beginning of treatment, began to give way to feelings of detachment, isolation, abject loneliness and hopelessness. An underlying bleak and often despairing emptiness became key features of the work, a depression which long preceded the sexually violent and exploitative world that engulfed her during the early adolescent years. Increasingly, she conveyed an internal world with little expectation that any of her emotional needs could be met.

At times, in desperation, she was keen to convince me that she had an idealised relationship with her mother, telling me how close they were and how 'they told each other everything'. She tried to convince me her mother, father, aunts and cousins all loved her and could look after her and that she was only taken away from them because she 'bunked from school'. She couldn't understand why she could not return to her home town, even at Xmas or for her birthday. The court had 'got it wrong'.

It would only be in the latter part of her second year of therapy that she could tell me a little about her mother's drinking and depression and how her father was involved with a new family and had little time for her. She gradually told me a little of the grooming aspect of the men's gang and how she and the other girls would be given phones as a means they could keep tabs on them. She felt other girls in the syndicate, though appearing loyal, would betray her at any time. She felt watched, monitored and controlled. She could acknowledge the feeling of being special, of being 'kept an eye on' and of 'being needed' by the gang even though the punishments and brutality, at times, were the pay off.

In her mind, I (or the staff on the unit) could become one of these figures who was suspect, rivalrous, controlling and mistrusted. In her paranoia, she felt I was gaining her trust to betray her and join forces with those who were out to blame her and punish her. This was in contrast to a much younger Jemma who longed to 'be kept an eye on' by caring and containing figures.

Further sessions indicated the extent to which she could withdraw into a nightmarish state of mind. These defensive structures were continuously brought to life through the interplay of the on-going disturbed relationships. These were mainly with a weak mother figure, the staff on the unit and, of course, me, her therapist, all of whom she believed wanted to control, dominate or exploit her. Alternatively, she experienced them as 'voyeurs' and helpless to help her. She mainly described a depressed, hostile, entangled relationship with females.

Her mind could become completely immersed in the rivalrous aspects of female relationships in such a way they seem to serve as a defensive retreat from making ordinary contact, not just with me in the room but with other aspects of her own functioning.

I began to wonder whether Jemma's early difficulties were compounded, possibly from the terror of feeling overwhelmed by un-metabolised parental projections, by withdrawing into a destructive internal organisation to protect herself. I have found Rosenfeld's (1971) description of an internal gang organisation, helpful in illustrating the predicament my patient finds herself in. He writes:

> The destructive narcissism of these patients often appears highly organised as if one were dealing with a powerful gang, dominated by a leader, who controls all the members of the gang ....
>
> *(Rosenfeld, 1971, p. 174)*

He highlights the tight grip it holds on other parts of the personality in order to maintain the 'status quo' in which:

> The main aim seems to be to prevent the weakening of the organisation and to control the members of the gang so they will not desert the destructive organisation and join the positive parts of the self or betray the secrets of the gang to the police, the protective superego, standing for the helpless analyst who might be able to save the patient.
>
> *(p. 174)*

Jemma eloquently describes the anguish of feeling a victim to this internal, gang-like regime which dominated the early phase of the therapeutic work. Her narratives depict an internal situation in which she can feel repeatedly controlled and exploited by others. In particular, she feels herself to be trapped in a primitive triangulation with a retaliatory mother figure and a seductive hostile father figure.

It is in the countertransference where I can feel powerfully gripped by, and can often feel helpless to, the gang-like projections. I can feel completely ignored and insignificant when my interpretations are jeered at or belittled when she would complain that she saw me as a lonely old lady who wanted to spoil her sexual potency, her capacity to attract men and excite them. She would mock and taunt me with accusations that I resented her youth and that I wanted to prevent her from what she most wished. That was to join, in unison, in an excited intercourse with the men whilst also telling me she had never been sexually exploited, had never had sex with older men and that it was the perversity of my mind and other professionals who had that idea in their minds.

However, when I did attempt to challenge her more robustly, she could identify with the tyrannical, possessive and controlling aspects of the regime she was so frightened of. In these moments, I think she conveys a core difficulty for her, in that she longs for 'partnership' and is momentarily able to act upon this by turning to me. She then becomes very frightened of a harsh and cruel superego figure that represents a very destructive aspect of herself. It attacks her own creative and productive inner life, as well as attacking any creative thinking links with me. In this way, it can feel that the analytic method itself is felt by Jemma to be a threat.

As I became aware of the double bind when a response or no response is an ineffective one, I began to see how subtly I can be invited to enact this sado-masochistic dynamic with her. I have found it a real struggle to differentiate from moment to moment when she is subtly and simultaneously projecting her infantile/child needy self into me whilst she moves into an identification with the bad object organisation and how quickly this situation is reversed if I refer to it. I increasingly saw that she created a reverse situation in the transference such that I felt myself to be in the position of a small child: helpless, feeling unable to make any meaningful impact or guilty because I felt that contact might make the situation worse. In fleeting moments, her defensive stance would break down, and she would momentarily cry out, "Why did my dad leave, why did my mum stop caring?" or "why did social services take so long to get me out of there?"

Through the countertransference experience, I think I began to understand more of the predicament she was in; of how she feels her own vulnerable distressed states provoke and disturb, what she feels is a very damaged maternal figure. It seems she remains caught up in a state of 'entanglement' with her mother's mind and struggles to differentiate between what is herself, what's her mother's mind and what are her mother's own bad objects. Therefore, she feels she struggles to separate from or mourn the attachments to these figures in order to sustain a link with her own libidinal desires. To separate from this damaged figure is felt to be a betrayal, and yet to stay is felt to be a death-like existence. The abandoning figure can lead the young adolescent girl into premature pseudo-adult sexuality as a means to find a way of reevoking early satisfactions of being held, caressed and attended to as an infant, but with damaging consequences.

Over time, held within the firm structures of the work (including social work and educational support), she began to introject a more thinking and reflective object, one that could begin to contain the overwhelming primitive terrors and anxieties linked to fears of abandonment. She could begin to develop a capacity to be aware of her own differing emotional states. This paralleled development in her capacity to think, be more reflective and, in school, she began to learn and passed some GCSE's.[2]

As she approached turning 18 years old, she wore professionals down by her relentless 'demands' to be 'moved on' from the semi-secure unit to a semi-independent unit (a pseudo-independent unit). Her wish for concrete evidence that she could 'move on' in her life was externalised. Unfortunately, when her wish to be moved was granted, she transferred to a semi-independent unit living with other vulnerable and disturbed young people with little adult support. She tried to continue to attend therapy, but within weeks, the excitement and delinquency of her new living situation drew her further away, and eventually, she stopped coming.

Even at the end of therapy, she still struggled to believe that I, or others trying to provide care for her, could receive and survive her projections and whether, as her therapist, I could be robust enough to survive her turning me into a cruel object that intrudes into her. Despite her fear of this toxicity, she had allowed, for brief periods of time, an experience of the work tolerating and surviving her anger and containing her more depressive anxieties. In turn, this has led her to increasingly taking in some good experiences and has increased her capacity to tolerate, though very tenuously, a degree of psychic pain.

Discussion

In thinking about Jemma's difficulties, it could be said that her earliest introjects, as an infant, were, in fact, her parents' hostile and damaged internal objects. For Jemma, there was always a failed or destructive parental figure in the therapy, one who was so preoccupied with their own disturbances that it created a situation in which there seemed to be little in the way of a parental mind for Jemma to project into. At times, she despaired as to whether she could get better because her objects couldn't get better. As a defence against what can feel like irreparable 'damage' both internally and externally, she took flight from the pain of her situation and took refuge in a world of excitement, one in which her contempt for any awareness of her own infantile vulnerability and need for care were often mocked.

Her difficulties in really acknowledging me, or of taking in my thoughts, led me to consider whether there was a tension between the 'desires' for and 'terror' of fusion with her objects, suggesting a denial of the space between us and a real failure of triangulation. This entanglement does not allow room for mourning the parental attachments of childhood and of separation and individuation.

Importantly (even if in a limited way), the therapeutic relationship can offer a space in which containment, thinking and integration can potentially begin to take place. Mourning the early loss of parental attachments (even disturbed ones) is essential in the work with these youngsters. The therapy structure and the capacity of the therapist to bear and feel the brunt of the failed parental projections are essential for these young girls to begin to introject a more robust containment in which mourning the attachments of childhood can begin to take place and which allows new relationships and development.

Notes

1 Jemma represents a composite of a number of adolescent girls I have seen in psychotherapeutic treatment in both in-patient and outpatient settings. They were all girls who had been groomed into sexually exploitative gangs. All had been removed from their families and were cared for by social services' provision.
2 GCEs are the standard General Certificate of Education examinations taken by teenagers in the UK (excluding Scotland)

References

Bion, W.R. (1962) A theory of thinking, in: Bion, W. *Second Thoughts: Selected Papers on Psychoanalysis*, 110–119. London: Karnac, 1984.

Britton, R. (1998) *Belief and Imagination: Explorations in Psychoanalysis*. London: Brunner-Routledge.

Bronstein, C. (2020) *Psychosis and psychotic functioning in adolescence. The International Journal of Psychoanalysis*. Vol. 101, no. 1, 136–151.

Freud, S. (1917) Mourning and melancholia, in: *Complete Works of Freud*, Standard Edition., 19:237–260. London: Hogarth.

Laufer, M. (1982) Developmental breakdown in adolescence. Problems of understanding and helping, in: Laufer, M. *Adolescence*, 9–16. Monograph 8. London: Brent Adolescent Centre.

Polmear, C. (2010) Dying to live: Mourning, melancholia and the adolescent process, Chapter. 3 in: McGinley E and Varchevker A. (eds) *Enduring Loss: Mourning Depression and Narcissism through the Life Cycle*. London & New York: Routledge Press.

Rosenfeld, H. (1971) *A clinical approach to the psychoanalytic theory of the life and death instincts: An investigation into the aggressive aspects of narcissism*. The International Journal of Psychoanalysis. Vol. 52, 169–178.

Tustin, F. (1990) *The Protective Shell in Children and Adults*. London: Karnac.

Williams, G. (1997) *Internal Landscapes and Foreign Bodies*. London: Duckworth.

3

CHILDREN HAVING CHILDREN

The cycle of exploitation in pregnancy and premature motherhood

Fiona Henderson

Wherever there is sexual exploitation between men and women, there will be pregnancies and children born. The contexts for this are much more varied and subtle than the commonly imagined scenario of an unwanted baby conceived by rape, although, of course, this is something that also happens. A baby may be central in a woman's wishful fantasy that an exploitative situation could be 'turned good' or that she could live 'happy ever after' with the baby's father. There may be siblings born to the same mother where the paternity of each, or some of them, is unknown or unclear. Confusion reigns in such families as the mother may feel differently about each child depending on her recollections or fantasies about how they were conceived. The shadow of an abusive man might hang around some children, while others are regarded in a more benign or even magical way. Massive splitting can come to dominate family life in an attempt to deny or simplify the complexities of the situation. Children can grow up in families that are shrouded in mystery and shame, sensing this but not understanding what it's about. They can come to feel identified with secrecy and shamefulness making them vulnerable to emotional problems later on such as depression or addictive states of mind.

How a woman understands her involvement in sexual exploitation will determine how well she can recover from the experience and go on developing capacities to keep herself and her children safe. This psychotherapeutic work will take a woman back to her early life with her own parents, remembered or imagined, in particular, how the parents' sexual and procreative relationship was internalised as a version of 'coming together' that necessarily excluded her. This Oedipal template for all subsequent relationships determines how able we are to register painful emotions like frustration, longing,

DOI: 10.4324/9781003020370-3

and exclusion and whether we can draw on parental figures to help us manage these powerful feelings in a sensitive way. Our Oedipal situation will go on to influence what we do with our adult bodies, as hunger that can't be tolerated is more likely to seek satisfaction in risky and compulsive ways. An association between craving and destructiveness in our emotional lives is an idea very familiar to psychoanalytic thinking (Riviere 1937; Bion 1959).

Every baby is born into the particular circumstances of its mother's Oedipal situation, real and imagined. The mother's internalised version of her own mother's body and its contents, and of her parents' original coupling, will play a large part in her desire, or lack of desire, for a baby. How a young girl has witnessed and fantasised about her mother's union with her father, or with other men, will influence how her own curiosities and longings evolve. The way a baby girl is physically handled and looked after lays the foundation for how she grows up to imagine herself within her body. In some women, traumatic intrusions across the body boundary, or into personal space, are lodged somatically as 'indigestible experiences', bypassing imagination and thought, then acted out concretely and compulsively through procedures like cosmetic surgery, self-mutilation, and attacks on the procreative self through repeated abortions or babies given up for adoption (Foster 2019).

The adolescent girl is pulled into an identification with her mother, or mother's body, as her sexuality matures, and this can reawaken earlier conflicts around separation and dependency. This process is fraught with ambivalence which may be acted out in perverse and harmful ways as the young woman tries to bring emotional turmoil under control. Pregnancy may be sought from a deep-seated need to be loved or to have something good inside; it may be 'procured' through sexual contact that is risky, exploitative, or unrewarding so that the baby arrives already bearing projections from its mother's own story. The pregnancy and birth can be both enactments and attempted solutions to profound trauma and loss (Raphael-Leff 1994). I recall working with a very disturbed woman who kept having babies she couldn't look after. One day she went to the corner shop to buy milk and 'came back pregnant', several days later, having bumped into a man known locally for exploiting vulnerable women. She was unable to explain how it had happened but conveyed a strong sense of now having got what she wanted despite everyone else's concern.

Adolescent girls can be drawn into sexual relationships prematurely as a way of using their bodies to re-evoke something of the earliest contact between mother and child, particularly where this has not been satisfying or satisfactory in actual life. It is often only fore-play that is welcomed, whereas penetration and emotional involvement with a sexual partner stir primitive anxieties of merger or falling apart. Sexual partners are not related to as real people with emotional needs, and the desire for contact is driven by a longing to return to an earlier state of primary omnipotence experienced as a baby, or even unborn baby; for these women, the birth of a real baby might be a calamity. (Pines 1993). The same pregnant woman I mentioned before, referred constantly to her 'baby tummy', conveying how she was now in the grip of a powerful identification with her unborn baby, merged, and as often happens, briefly stabilised by this blissful state of narcissistic gratification.

A woman might have a baby, unconsciously, to repair a sense of deprivation in herself. Her identity can become confused with that of the baby, leading to problems as the baby's individuality starts to be felt. Early or repeated pregnancies may be a woman's attempt to create a version of mother and baby that has been missing or longed for in herself. However, this attempted solution might also be an expression of rage about what hasn't been right or even good enough; an act of revenge, by exploiting her body and repeatedly 'giving away' the babies that come from it, perhaps as she feels her mother did with her.

Social workers are familiar with mothers and babies who seem well bonded during the first few months before things start to fall apart as the baby's capacities and interests grow. The mother may have provided for her baby on a practical level, but something more subtle and relational may be missing or disturbed. An insecure mother, who enjoyed the feeling of her baby being dependent on her in the early weeks, might now feel rejected and resentful as her baby starts to look around. Sometimes, we can see this painfully enacted when a mother tries to 'catch' her baby's gaze by imposing her face in the baby's line of sight or by physically moving the baby's head towards her. It is as if the baby's growing curiosity is felt as a kind of turning away, re-evoking earlier experiences of rejection, impenetrability, or neglect.

An adhesive or enmeshed attachment style can look like a mother attending to her baby's every need, keeping the baby close, but in fact, this entangled situation, based on projective identification, confuses the baby's dependency needs with the mother's own infantile cravings and deprivation. There is denial of separation and difference. When the reality of individuation begins to emerge, a disturbed mother might respond with harshness, paranoid outbursts, or a more subtle withdrawal from her baby by neglecting the baby's needs or starting to imagine a new pregnancy.

During an assessment, I watched a mother bounce her baby on her chest; the baby squealed with what seemed to be a precarious kind of delight. At one point, the baby's foot tapped against his mother's body, in an ordinary way, due to all the jiggling about. The mother sprung back, outraged, exclaiming: 'you fucking kicking me, or what!' before handing the baby over to his father. This mother was not able to use her baby's gesture as an opening for communicative contact and play, an opportunity for discovery and learning. We can see how an insecure or persecuted mother might interpret her baby's ordinary moves in a paranoid way, leaving the baby vulnerable to harm, misunderstanding, or neglect.

Young women who have borderline or narcissistic difficulties are particularly susceptible to the kind of trauma and coercion that characterise sexually exploitative experiences. Feelings of emptiness and low self-worth in the women are perpetuated by constant fear of abandonment or exclusion by others, including, of course, the men who exploit. Pregnancy provides a brief respite from these unbearable anxieties and longings because it fills the body with life, and provides the mother with a fantasy of an object that is totally dependent on her in a way that is only ever gratifying – static, non-developmental, a perfect fit, and a narcissistic extension of herself – and quite different from the reality of a dependent baby who is demanding, perplexing, apparently greedy and unsatisfied, striving for independence, constantly changing, and interested in other people and things beyond mother.

A pregnant woman with borderline difficulties can feel intensely identified with her pregnant body or unborn baby in a way that can become a psychic retreat; a defensive structure in the mind designed to avoid emotional pain (Steiner 1993). Such preoccupation with her 'baby tummy' can have the quality of an 'elopement', a secretive, self-contained state of running away from realities and responsibilities such as other children, or from guilt about what happened to previous babies. It can be misunderstood as appropriate maternal preoccupation in pregnancy when, in fact, it has a different and more delusional quality. This can be an important distinction to discover when assessing risk, and it involves noticing *how* a woman talks about her pregnancy and whether she conveys a sense of perspective where she can also think about her existing children and her wider life.

One of the difficulties for child protection work is that the risks to newborn babies often go unseen because of the more hidden and perverse nature of dynamics that can lead to harm. There are cases where young children are removed from home due to parenting concerns, but a newborn baby stays at home with mum, as if nothing worrying can be happening to an infant this early on. This is where it is important to become familiar with features of mother-infant interaction that are concerning and to be aware of our tendency, or wish, to view mothers and babies in a sentimental or rose-tinted way. All the while, we need to keep in mind that every mother has unmet, infantile needs of her own, which she will be more or less able to suspend in the interests of looking after her baby. The importance of child-centredness can be misinterpreted by family services, including family courts, in a way that contributes to further neglect of the 'child-within' the parent, especially when that adult is presenting risk or harm. Sometimes, parents can feel that the whole system is preoccupied with their child, leaving them, and their emotional needs, out of sight. It is by talking to parents about the childlike aspects of themselves that we help adults develop a keener sensitivity to the emotional lives of their children. This is often the focus of psychotherapy with parents, sometimes 'prescribed' as a condition of care or contact agreements, but I would argue that it should also form the backdrop of all interventions with families where there are concerns about children's safety and wellbeing.

I worked for many years as a psychotherapist linked to child protection teams and the family court. I have been interested in how therapy can help women understand the more destructive aspects of themselves as partners and as parents, and how this harmfulness connects up with their own individual stories. What might progress involve for these women; what's at stake in moving forward, and how can professionals feel more confident about a mother's care of her children? This is painful and difficult psychotherapeutic work for women who are raising concerns, especially when there are deep-seated insecurities which make it hard to hold on to trust. Progress is usually 'one step forward, several back' because helpful steps towards understanding are often followed by rebounds into heightened anxiety and acting out. When the therapy has been recommended or ordered by the professional network, there is the ever-present clock ticking in the background, compelling the work unrealistically 'within the timeframe of the child', and creating a climate of scrutiny around a process that requires privacy and trust at the best of times. Many therapists are reluctant to work with clients who have been 'sent' because of a belief that the client has to move some way, by themselves, 'towards the object' in order to mobilise a healthy concern and desire for change within themselves, however small or fragile that might be.

I sometimes think about the family court, and its jurisdiction, as having a 'paternal function' in the psychoanalytic sense of setting limits and conditions and standing firm by the realities of appropriateness and time. We might surmise that parents will differ in their response to such paternalism depending on their early experiences of authority figures in the past. Whether they experience the judge as protective or persecutory will influence how they engage with the recommendations and requirements that ensue. For example, some women become pregnant during care proceedings concerning their other children. Instead of engaging with the seriousness of these proceedings, facing up to what has not been possible or right, the mother takes matters into her own hands, and replaces the baby that might be taken from her, triumphing over the object, and the system, that controls, torments and ultimately abandons her. She does the very thing that no one wants her to do and often keeps the pregnancy undisclosed, like a kind of 'trump card', until the point when it will have the greatest effect; a moment of revenge to lift her from awareness of unbearable guilt and loss. These mothers used to be known colloquially as 'frequent fliers', which was rather apt if we think about the function of their pregnancies as a manic flight from loss, emptiness, and responsibility. It can be important to help these women work with the very professionals they identify to be the problem; to face their hostility more directly rather than repeatedly acting it out.

Alternatively, the court process and child protection team can be experienced in a more benign way as coming together with parents to problem-solve their difficulties and support them through necessary change. This system of 'therapeutic justice' has been developed in the United Kingdom by The Family Drug and Alcohol Court (Bambrough, Crichton and Webb 2019), which has worked successfully with 'end of the road' families to break cycles of intergenerational trauma and abuse. This more integrated, less adversarial, way of engaging troubled families provides a healthy model of Oedipal relationships, where parents can think together about their children's needs, and a child can begin to tolerate being seen and thought about by others (Britton 1989).

The case I will discuss is one in which I became a new kind of parental figure to a young mother who came into psychotherapy with me; someone who could involve her more actively in determining what the safeguarding network should know while not side-stepping the seriousness of the concerns, and a therapist-parent who could work collaboratively with 'the other parent' network to stand firm by the established facts, while also insisting upon privacy and respect while the client worked on her difficulties and herself. This is the case of a young woman involved in an exploitative and coercive relationship with a violent man over many years. The relationship led to the birth of three children, all of whom had been removed into kinship care.

Nina's journey into therapy

Nina was twenty-three years old when I met her. By the time she was twenty, all three of her children had been placed with relatives on both maternal and paternal sides; her eldest daughter at the age of eight, and her younger daughter and son at two weeks old and at birth, respectively. Social services had been keeping an eye on the family for years as the children's father was well known for violent crime. Nina lived alone at an undisclosed address, having left an eight-year relationship with this man after her third child was removed into care. Supervised contact with the children was conditional on Nina remaining out of touch with their father.

As I came to understand, Nina's early history made her vulnerable to hooking up with an exploitative partner. She carried emotional wounds and unmet needs that would draw her into relationships offering a certain kind of attention and perverse version of care. Throughout childhood, Nina's mother had tantalised and tormented her by being alluring and impermeable at the same time. One minute Nina was 'Mummy's little princess, dressed up like Mummy and prematurely sexualised, while the next minute, she was painfully abandoned or alone, as her mother failed to notice her or didn't respond to her distress. Later, during her teens, her mother often seemed provoked by her into furious rages or cruel attacks. Nina wondered whether her mother was jealous of her, but she couldn't imagine how this might be the case. Her own self-esteem was so fragile that she relied on doing her mother's bidding which often got her into fights.

Nina had learned about the psychotherapy service from other mothers at court; she had looked it up online and pushed hard with her general practitioner to be referred. 'This is my last chance saloon', she told me when we first met, 'doing two years here is what they want, so you can get your kids back after'. She viewed the service as a detention centre of sorts, where she would 'do her time' to the satisfaction of the local authority and the family court. She showed little curiosity about where she actually was, or any real sense that she wanted, or needed, to be understood. She seemed to have an idea that just turning up would be enough as if she was seeking a kind of pardon, or exoneration perhaps, although this changed in noticeable ways as the work progressed. It was interesting, however, that the therapy had not been 'prescribed' by the authorities at court. She had happened upon it by herself and made an effort to get referred; in retrospect, I thought this was an important factor in how able she was to put the opportunity to use.

On the face of it, Nina was not a hopeful psychotherapy case. I thought that if I took her on, I would need to keep her file in the 'bottom drawer' of my desk where questions would not be asked. I later linked this reaction to the projections of 'no hoper' that women like Nina often attract, where something hidden and shameful gets internalised by them, perpetuating vicious cycles of deprivation and harm. There was also the constant threat of intrusion into the work by the child protection team, 'camped outside the door', eagerly awaiting results.

Nina was preoccupied with battling social workers to prove her competence as a mother. She had little to say about why people were concerned but mentioned, in passing, being easily provoked to anger, just like her mother, and feeling constantly on guard. She had a lively intelligence, and I thought she was at risk of misusing it to prop up an aggrieved state of mind that damaged her relationships with professionals and held her progress back. I wanted to give her some time, without judgement, to see if she could slow down enough to think. In hindsight, she came to the psychotherapy service full of bluster when, actually, she craved a place to land where she would be recognised as herself. She quickly appreciated the 'grown-up-ness' of this adult mental health service which was offering her a chance to grow.

Nina's case mobilised competing agendas: her own wish for reprieve from cruel judgement from outside; her social worker's demand, unstated, that I reform this 'failed mother' for society's sake; and my own hope that I could help Nina understand herself better so that she might engage, more effectively, with her child protection team. My work with Nina often stirred dissatisfaction in one side or the other. At times, I could sense the local authority desperate to intrude into the private space of the therapy, understandably impatient to 'know' whether and when this young mother could be transformed. At other times,

I would feel abandoned, in the isolation of the consulting room, to perform some kind of miracle so that everyone else could relax. Nina had never been shown ordinary privacy or boundaries, and so, by protecting the therapeutic frame, I hoped to give her a new experience that would help her become more trusting and more interested in her emotional life.

At first, Nina was terrified that I would team up with the network against her and bring the therapy to an abrupt end. This was a fantasy based on repeated experiences of having good things sabotaged or taken away. There were memories of violent exchanges between her parents which she could hear but not properly see. Later, when her mother had a succession of part-ners, Nina always felt that she was in the way. Nina was surprised that instead, I teamed up with her to think about our connection with the profes-sionals involved in her case. What would she like people to know, and how were they going to hear? This was a turning point in our work; for the first time, it seemed, someone was helping her direct her own progress rather than enviously or spitefully standing in her way.

Settling into the work

At the start of therapy, Nina commented on the 'homeliness' of my room, ex-claiming, 'Oh, it's lovely and warm in here'. Some weeks on, she found it sur-prising that I had no decorations up for Christmas, unlike 'all the excitement in Reception and outside'. These reactions to the setting mirrored fluctua-tions in Nina's relationship with me where, sometimes, she was pleased she could talk honestly, without feeling judged, while at other times, she found the therapy, and me, overly serious, strange, and unconnected to real life.

Her way of talking about herself didn't always make sense, and she would exaggerate or invent things seemingly for effect. She linked this to 'dyslexia which was never picked up at school', but I think it was also a way in which she tried to manage the fragmented state of her mind, the shards of memories, the faint aspirations; like weaving a net of stories to hold herself together. For example, she had an abiding memory of her father taking her to his pub as a young girl, where she sat happily under the table; 'after that I never saw him again'. Similarly, she told me, 'I'm studying law to be a barrister in the fam-ily court'. It transpired that she could barely read or write and was working hard to remedy this through evening classes. These half-truths were impor-tant to Nina, to be treated with genuine interest rather than scepticism. They were also embellishments of sorts, propping up a fragile self-esteem.

Nina came to sessions 'dolled up' in sophisticated clothes which made her look older than her years and yet vulnerable as well. Underneath the fake fur coat, she wore flimsy, revealing garments despite the weather which was often cold. Her face was heavily made-up, and she worked hard not to let her mascara run if she almost cried. Some time into therapy she removed the extensions from her hair. She had been her mother's rag doll for years, she said, and now she wanted to be more herself. She took up judo, which she was good at, and started wearing androgynous sports clothes most of the time. I thought she was now attracted to a more contained form of combat from the uncontained violence she had witnessed growing up.

Nina's progress in therapy was fragile, and helpful sessions were often followed by manic and grandiose activity, 'putting her world to rights', or by a return to denial and an aggrieved state of mind, both of which made it harder to connect with her. She would try to resolve things with her mother overnight, demand meetings with the network, and file applications to court. Her capacity to look honestly at herself during sessions was fleeting and quickly eclipsed by concrete justifications to 'set the record straight'. Her need to prove herself in everyone's eyes often made it hard to stay with painful feelings for long. She wanted to believe that she was changing more quickly and easily than she actually was and that the seriousness of what needed to be faced could be played down or denied. These kinds of common and powerful defence can also influence professional teams, leading them to become unrealistically hopeful about a client's progress.

Intergenerational factors

Family culture played a key part in understanding Nina's case. She came from an area of England where generations often lived together, or close by, and traditional roles prevailed, with women holding sway in the home. She grew up first in her mother's house and then with her maternal grandparents around the corner. Although she now had a council flat of her own, she still regarded her grandparents' house as home, and shuttled back and forth between these places, retracing her journey from adolescence to adulthood, over and over again. Nina's grandparents were very important to her, having largely brought her up. Now they were raising her eldest daughter who had been placed with them after removal from her care. Nina's mother also spent a lot of time at her parent's house, and it seemed that this was the one stable, intact home which held the family together but from which no one could ever properly move on.

Nina's family was a large, entangled group of women – grandmother, mother, and aunts – described as constantly bickering, vying with each other, and whipping up exaggerated dramas. Spiteful exchanges were common, and there seemed to be no loyalty or capacity for concern. The women were sensitive to feeling excluded and so there was a tendency to intrude. Nina's phone would constantly go off during sessions creating the impression that she was always in the midst of a family saga, very often her own. The few men in Nina's family had tried, through the generations, to moderate this heightened emotion, but it seemed that they, too, were at the mercy of the women's demands. Unemployment and poor physical health had left its mark, but these men, especially Nina's grandfather, seemed to be appreciated as a containing, stable backdrop.

Nina's relationship with her mother was often on her mind. She never felt properly recognised in her mother's eyes, always sensing her mother's preoccupation with herself. Precocious sexuality was a way of satisfying unfulfilled longings for contact with her mother, but it also stirred unbearable anxieties about being taken over or destroyed. Having a baby in her early teens was Nina's attempt, unconsciously, to forge a link with her mum, who was experienced both as possessively controlling and largely taken up with herself. Her mother was unsupportive, and school was more helpful at the time. 'There was a special scheme' she told me proudly, 'which let us bring our babies into school'. Nina went on to be closer to this first child than to her other two, which I think is partly because the school provided a home for the baby and her in this way.

Soon after Nina's first baby was born, Nina's mother became pregnant by a man she had recently met. Nina felt her mum could not allow her to have anything good without expecting the same for herself; once again, competing with her for the limelight. In the course of therapy, Nina started to become more interested in her mother's own predicament growing up. She recalled her mother's memory of sitting on the doorstep as a girl, waiting for her dad to come home from work to relieve the claustrophobic atmosphere in the house. In Nina's family, girls were closer to their grandmothers than their mothers; perhaps because this offered more breathing space from rivalry and intrusion. Mothers struggled to be affectionate to daughters as they, too, were at the mercy of powerful identifications and unacknowledged ambivalence.

Fear of loss or sabotage

Nina held a deep-seated fear that good or longed for things would be taken away. She linked this to the early loss of her father which she experienced in Oedipal terms as mother having driven him away due to envy of Nina's love for him. She felt the loss of her father very keenly, but I thought it was the primary loss, or 'never gain', of her mother that underpinned Nina's difficulties now. Nina's 'giving up' her own babies into care could be understood as an unconscious acting out of her own mother's early rejecting-neglecting of her. It also enacted an omnipotent, masochistic denial of the goodness within herself and her own babies' need of this. Nina had tremendous difficulty believing that she had good and nourishing things inside her. Her focus was on external appearances, victory, and triumph rather than hard won achievement. Nina's mother could be enviously cruel and spoiling. Destructive rivalry between mother and daughter was always close to the surface and regularly erupted around new grievances. Nina described how her mother recently had a 'boob job' and then spoke resentfully about the unfairness of Nina's perfect figure while she 'had to pay'. In therapy, Nina worked on her preoccupation with this kind of persecution to think more about her own difficulty in protecting what was important in her life, most notably her struggle to protect her children from her own envy and destructiveness.

Fear of getting messed up

Nina kept a spotless home. She used housework as a way of discharging anger and anxiety and to help her feel that she was putting her world to rights. She found it unbearable when friends sat on her sofa and moved her scatter cushions about, and she would struggle to resist an urge to rearrange them immediately. In a similar way, she would try to tidy up any internal disturbance caused by the therapy, or me, by 'getting to work' on what had been revealed or learnt. It was hard to imagine that she could make room for the messiness of children in her immaculate life. Similarly, her sexuality seemed to be closed down, or inaccessible, and she spoke as if she had no sexual imagination or desire. As time went on, Nina started to question her preoccupation with external appearances, and this opened up greater interest in her emotional life. She came to sessions more casually dressed or with lighter makeup on her face. Towards the end of our work, Nina met a man who she liked, and I was able to see the full extent of her anxiety about letting someone in.

Too close or too far

There was a constant push and pull in Nina's mind between relationships feeling too close or too far apart. If she let people get to know her, she worried that they would try to take her over. Conversely, she often felt over-looked or excluded by others and she struggled to make friends. Nina suffered from asthma, and after some months in therapy, she commented that her throat was not as tight, and she felt there was more room inside her body. She struggled to express strong or angry feelings to me out of fear that if I was in her direct firing line, I would turn her away. She imagined that she had been conceived by warring parents and that she was the cause of ongoing conflict in the wider family. In time, she came to see how much she needed to find a manageable way of interacting with her family which allowed her space to breathe and think.

Nina had no experience of emotional containment by her mother, and she was totally unused to someone being alongside her without competing or intruding. She struggled to use her own mind to help her manage difficult feelings, having never had an object that could really think about her. During the therapy, her memories of childhood started to become more 'fleshed out'. Her nightmares, which had often been about intrusion, decreased in frequency, and when she did have one, she came to her senses more easily than before, feeling less compelled to check around the house. This showed an increase in her capacity to reflect and to bring reality to bear upon her unconscious life.

Nina found the pace of therapy frustrating, and she had an unrealistic idea of why she needed to come. As she started to understand more about her difficulties, she seemed less persecuted by the changes going on inside her and more able to see therapy as an unfolding process which would not necessarily make everything better. This paved the way for the work of mourning what she had not been able to experience either as a child herself, or with her own children, and the reality of what she had lost. She started to understand, painfully, that she needed to sacrifice certain things – such as unrealistic strivings – in order to safeguard the progress she was making, and she began to talk about her wish to have a secure relationship before knowing whether there might be future babies.

Keeping both mother and child in mind

While working with Nina, I was very aware of the importance of her family whom I would never meet, and in particular, her children. Nina was helped by coming on her own steam and being given time and space to think about herself as both a child and a parent. My involvement with Nina's children, through Nina's own voice, was essential in forging a therapeutic link with her. We often problem-solved emerging dilemmas about supervised contact or about the children's developmental struggles. Nina was proud to tell me about teaching her daughter to swim, away from the forensic glare of social services, as she would see it. We thought about birthday presents and how to handle tensions during contact, which was supervised by her grandmother and often gate-crashed, unhelpfully, by her mother. Through this careful balancing of focus, internal conflict between Nina's own emotional needs and those of her children started to ease, allowing her more opportunity to view herself as her children's mother, and to engage more directly with the responsibilities that this entailed.

My work with young mothers like Nina has left me with a question about child centred practice. I wonder whether our interpretation of this guiding principle, to promote and protect the needs and views of children, can at times play into splits that exist between adult and child services in a way that is picked up by parents who have histories of neglect, and who are desperate for recognition and a listening ear. In our concern, rightly, to attend to the voice of the child, we can find ourselves inadvertently shutting mothers out or not considering the stories of their own childhoods. These women often struggle with unconscious rivalry with their babies for care and attention, as giving birth stirs infantile longings to be mothered themselves. Identification with the new baby can have a narcissistic quality where the baby is experienced as greedily devouring all the goodies that are around. Nina described the generations of women in her family as envious and grasping. She worried about provoking envy in others as a way of masking the extent of deprivation she struggled with underneath. Perhaps it felt too risky to have anything really good for herself.

There is also the possibility that we get caught up engaging with mothers whose hunger for attuned contact overwhelms us to the point where we lose sight of the child (Harvey 2010). Winnicott's much quoted remark that 'there is no such thing as an infant' reminds us that no young child exists without maternal care (Winnicott 1960). I think that we need to approach our child centred practice always with the parent-child relationship in mind, even if the parent is physically out of the picture or is presenting cause for concern. It is noticeable that in adult mental health services, we tend to overlook the parent in our adult patients unless they bring this as a focus themselves. Child protection services, under constant pressure to identify risk, can become suffused with hostility and suspicion towards parents, even in the most subtle forms. These splits get played out between professionals, too, and deprived young parents are particularly vulnerable to falling down the gap that still exists between child and adult teams.

Addressing complexity

My work with mothers who are caught up in cycles of exploitation and whose children have been removed leads me to think that prevailing models underlying many therapeutic approaches are too simplistic. There is often a focus on 'trauma' in an undefined way, as if the nature, origin, and expression of that trauma are understandable and clear. The women are regarded, too narrowly, as victims of painful or damaging circumstances which have left them beyond responsibility and regret. This plays into splits already active in the women's internal worlds. Splits keep complexity at bay and organise perception into good and bad. Adverse experiences certainly feature in these women's lives. But the goal of therapy needs to be an understanding of how they are affected by these experiences now. This work extends beyond notions of victimhood into looking at one's own role in disturbance, both at the time and in how what happened has been carried forward in the mind, and in the way one engages with life.

Young women who have become caught-up in sexual exploitation have done so for complex reasons that need to be explored and understood. Hidden and addictive feelings like triumph, envy, and arousal have played a part in why the exploitative contact has continued. If therapy is to make a lasting difference, then these half-remembered feelings and sensations need to be explored, as well as the shame and guilt which exploited young adults so often carry. As practitioners, it can be difficult for us to think about a mother's misuse of her body or baby as a perverse or aggressive act. She is able to 're-create the destructive patterns of her own birth and childhood, inhabiting a domain within which she has power, where she can wreak vengeance and gain compensation for her own abuse and deprivation' (Motz 2008, p. 23). This retaliatory violence, conscious or unknown, can find itself communicated through the way a client interacts with the safeguarding network around her and her children. The client can start to feel that it is the professional network that exploits and abuses her in a depressing repetition of where she has been before.

Like other mothers in this situation, Nina was fired up by her case and by feuding with professionals in a way that seemed to hold her together and distance her from feelings of regret or grief. She believed she was born into the middle of a feud between her parents. She recalled early memories of them fighting at home, being unable to see them, but hearing the violent exchange. Later, she was often recruited to do her mother's bidding. 'Mummy's little Rottweiler', she called this aggressive aspect of herself that we got to know in therapy. To some extent, her mother's violence became libidinalised for Nina at an early age, a sexualised form of aggression, to manage her loneliness and terror about what was going on. As an adolescent, she was drawn into relationships with men with whom she could re-create this violent intercourse. The pregnancies that arose from this coupling were suffused with violent associations, and, in an unconscious pact with her perversion, Nina was unable, or unwilling, to protect the newborn babies from harm.

These powerful and disturbing dynamics lie at the heart of maternal abuse. At some stage in therapeutic work, these women will need help to make sense of how such destructive patterns have affected their lives and those of their children, ideally by exploring this disturbance as it emerges in the transference. Nina's anger and aggression were hard to get hold of during sessions. When she was upset, she tended to stay away and would wait until I came 'to find her' in a letter. On returning, she would have 'made up her face' again, and her disturbance would be out of reach. My sense was that Nina needed to protect me from the direct firing line of her aggression due to fear that I would turn her out. She knew that she needed this kind of help but had so little experience of people who could take her in, that she could only extremely tentatively begin to approach her feelings towards me. Later, she was able to talk about how stirred up she could feel after sessions, to an extent that was sometimes unbearable.

Loss, deprivation, and mourning

We cannot assume that mothers with early histories like Nina's are able to mourn the loss of pregnancies and children. The emotional work of mourning requires recognition of the ways in which one has acted destructively towards the same people and things that one has now lost. In other words, for these mothers, it depends on their capacity to think about what they bring to the story of losing their child, and its connection to the childhood that they lost themselves. Many of these mothers are preoccupied with a sense of grievance about their child's removal, such that they struggle to feel any concern for the part that they might have played or any wish to repair or make up for damage done. Nina talked very little about her pregnancies or what losing the children meant to her. She remained evasive about the violence in her relationship with their father until near the end when she started to describe clear victimisation through coercive control. I think the deep sense of shame she felt about 'failing' as a mother was somehow easier for her to tolerate than opening herself up to grief.

I recall a woman I assessed for court. Many years earlier, her baby had been removed at birth and now she was pregnant again. There was a lot of concern around. The woman cried in the assessment as she described having always carried a deep sense of agonising regret that she had never bathed her baby before giving him up. There was a faint hint of complaint – that she had been denied this 'right' before the baby had been snatched away – but the real sadness conveyed was that she had not had this chance to say goodbye. I thought about last rites and the importance of such rituals in the mourning process. Bathing a body allows recognition of that person's separateness from oneself and, therefore, challenges fantasies of omnipotent control. This mother's regret was a vital precursor to her longing for a new chance and something she could now think about with me in a very moving way.

Another woman I met for assessment described how she and her sister would go out at night to meet up with exploitative men. She remembered feeling triumph and contempt towards her parents as they sat in front of the television, barely raising their heads to inquire what time the girls would be back. This woman recalled a childhood that was profoundly lacking in ordinary parental care. There was something utterly tragic in how she conveyed the way she, half-knowingly, substituted chronic neglect for a fantasy of 'V.I.P attention' – being driven around 'in limousines', plied with alcohol and cigarettes, 'whatever you want Princess' – while being passed from one group of men to another in what amounted to organised rape. Her excitement and glee came to life again in the telling; a reminder of the powerful hold these dynamic processes have on the mind.

Realistic timeframes

Where there is a safeguarding network around these families, there will often be a question about whether the mother can be helped therapeutically within a timeframe that meets the needs of children who has been removed from her care or, indeed, any future children. This question often drives the pace of therapy unrealistically or obstructs frank discussion with the mother about what is, and is not, going to be possible at this point in time. It is more helpful to women who have had children removed if, in therapy, we can suspend any focus on getting lost children back and move the work into the arena of developing a capacity to parent safely in the future. This challenges the persecutory anxiety of 'them and us' or 'pass and fail' and takes a more developmental approach, helping women with troubled histories to grow emotionally through learning from experience, and reducing the panic and urgency which can pervade safeguarding teams and get into the therapeutic work.

Nina's therapy was undoubtedly too short. She needed longer than the one year I was able to give her in a publicly funded service. But it was a step towards Nina understanding herself better, beneath the make-up, so that she could engage more effectively with the network involved in her case, making them more aware of her vulnerabilities, and taking some of the persecutory heat out of relationships with those who were trying to help. The ending was felt as premature and painful, and Nina struggled to complain for fear that this would be interpreted as bad behaviour, lessening her chances of getting the further help she knew she desperately needed. She recalled her mother belittling her for wanting comfort and affection as a child, and also a feeling that mother had derived satisfaction from saying that Nina mattered less to her than her other children. She felt that I was showing her the door and that she would now be back in the hands of a safeguarding system that would barely acknowledge that it knew her, let alone recognise her needs. She planned to ask for further psychotherapy in due course but feared that other, more appreciated, clients would have taken her place.

Conclusion

Women who become pregnant from relationships of exploitation are enacting a cycle of deprivation, risk-taking, and abuse that repeats down the generations. Like so many others, Nina lacked experience of sensitive and reliable containment by a parental figure who could take her in and help her interpret and cope with the turmoil of her early emotional life. Therefore, it is unsurprising that as soon as she was able, Nina gravitated towards contact with men that seemed to offer special attention, love, and understanding. Of course, the warning signs are always there – these men are disturbed themselves, and violence and threat are never out of sight – but women like Nina are blinded by hunger, even for a perverse version of care, and they find it impossible to leave these men. They are unconsciously compelled to go on repeating painful and destructive dynamics from their past.

Pregnancies and babies may ensue in a seemingly haphazard way, but the unconscious phantasies propelling them were laid down by deep-seated deprivations from a previous time.

What we see is a cycle of emotional craving and dangerous acting out which needs to be understood as part of any successful intervention if we are to keep in mind the next generation who are at risk. The complex dynamics involved in how and why these babies are conceived underpins disturbed patterns of mothering where practical care may be adequate while more subtle, relational areas of care are distorted or lacking altogether. Furthermore, the powerful, addictive pull back into exploitation, where destruction goes on being repeated rather than recognised and worked through, leads some women to engage with safeguarding professionals in an untrustworthy or deceptive way.

For our part, as practitioners, in time-limited work, we often run the risk of making matters worse. Like most of these young mothers, Nina's experience of parental figures had been one of unreliability and rupture throughout her life. Therapeutic interventions that fail to acknowledge and address this reality, risk replaying an experience of premature abandonment, compounding chronic disillusionment with so-called 'help'. If we can notice and try to understand what is evoked by the process of ending, then we can enable women like Nina to face feelings of rage, responsibility, and loss head on, in a thoughtful way, including protest and complaint, echoes of earlier grief that was never heard. Such important psychological work can pave the way for a capacity to mourn one's own ruined childhood, one's children lost to care, and to dare to long for another chance.

References

Bambrough S, Crichton N and Webb S (2019) '*Better outcomes and better justice*', in A. Foster (ed.) *Mothers Accused and Abused. Addressing Complex Psychological Needs*. London: Routledge, pp. 125–137.

Bion WR (1959) *Attacks on linking*. International Journal of Psychoanalysis 40: 308–315. Also in: *Second Thoughts. Selected Papers on Psychoanalysis*. London: Heinemann, 1967; reprinted London: Karnac, 1984.

Britton R (1989) '*The missing link: Parental sexuality in the Oedipus complex*', in R. Britton, M. Feldman, E. O'Shaughnessy, & J. Steiner (eds.) *The Oedipus Complex Today: Clinical Implications*. London: Karnac, pp. 83–101.

Foster A (ed.) (2019) *Mothers Accused and Abused. Addressing Complex Psychological Needs*. London: Routledge.

Harvey A (2010) *Getting a grip on social work*. Journal of Social Work Practice 24:2, 139–153.

Motz A (2008) *The Psychology of Female Violence. Crimes against the Body*. London: Routledge.

Pines, D (1993) *A Woman's Unconscious Use of Her Body*. London: Virago.

Raphael-Leff J (1994) *'Imaginative bodies of childbearing'*, in A. Erskine & D. Judd (eds.) *The Imaginative Body. Psychodynamic Therapy in Health Care.* London: Whurr.

Riviere J (1937) *'Public lectures: Hate, greed, and aggression'*, in A. Hughes (ed.) *The Inner World and Joan Riviere.* London: Karnac, 1991.

Steiner J (1993) *Psychic Retreats: Pathological Organisations in Psychotic, Neurotic and Borderline Patients.* London: Routledge.

Winnicott DW (1960) *The theory of the parent-infant relationship.* International Journal of Psychoanalysis 41: 585–595.

4

UNDERSTANDING THE SIGNIFICANCE AND FUNCTION OF PROTECTIVE AGGRESSION IN CLINICAL WORK WITH YOUNG PEOPLE WHO WERE GROOMED AND SEXUALLY ABUSED

Ariel Nathanson

In her paper "comments on aggression" (1972), Anna Freud describes its infantile origins, ordinary development, and expression (Freud, 1972). She defines aggression as primarily a drive, although she acknowledges that it might also be seen as an ego capacity. As a drive it is innate, similar to the libido. It has its impetus, the relief when it is expressed and the inevitable distress if it is blocked. As a capacity it is learned from experience, mediated by the ego, and used in the creation of the capacity to protect the self from harm.

Interpreting my patients' experiences, I believe that the absence of protective aggression, its inhibition or perversion, is central to the trauma of grooming and abuse. Restoring protective aggression or developing it in cases of early inhibition is therefore crucial to treatment and recovery.

As suggested by Anna Freud, the capacity for aggression is learned from experience. As such, it is relational, environmentally dependent, and susceptible to trauma and other relational influences. I would imagine that it is also impacted by the wider culture, gender, and race relations. Racism, for example, is a good example for a perversion of aggression, and being a chronic victim of it might have a huge impact on the way a sense of aggression internally develops as a benign protective capacity.

All these environmental-relational experiences from the personal to the wider cultural, contribute to the creation of a capacity to experience aggression as benign and protective. When the link between aggression and protection is severed by relational trauma, a real sense of safety becomes very difficult to achieve. As a result, as many of my patients report and show, aggression is likely to be either inhibited or expressed in a variety of other ways, often creating cycles of harmful and addictive behaviours.

DOI: 10.4324/9781003020370-4

Grooming is commonly known as the time in which a perpetrator gains the confidence and trust of his victim in order to abuse and exploit them later. I believe that grooming can be seen from a much wider perspective to include all relational experiences in which protective aggression is being hacked into and, as a result, suspended, misdirected, inhibited, or perverted.

In this chapter, I analyse my patients' experiences to describe how grooming as a relational experience interferes with the development and use of protective aggression. In doing so, I adopt both a perpetrator and victim's perspective. I then turn to explore the psychodynamic significance of grooming in clinical work and how restoring a sense of protective aggression is crucial to recovery.

The clinical material I have used here is based on what I have heard and learned from my patients. However, the histories and general experiences are presented as an amalgamation of profiles that amount to what might be considered as a presentation that would fit the experience of many young people who were groomed and abused.

Grooming

The grooming stage in sexual abuse is the time perpetrators gradually use their aggression in a perverse way, and victims start losing their capacity to use their aggression to protect themselves.

A patient once described his grooming experience as the slow mixing-in of a dark cordial into his relationship to a trusted older cousin who he admired. The toxic cordial is a fantastic metaphor to describe any attack in which the loss of power to resist is experienced gradually. Indeed, this patient remembered an experience many others have conveyed in other ways; intrusions were subtle and noticeable only after they already happened. For example, when his cousin showed him pornography, he saw the images before he had a chance to think about it, not to mention not having the capacity to fully appreciate and think about what he was being exposed to. When his cousin later touched him whilst they were watching pornography together, he noticed his cousin's hand on his body once the boundary had been breached, never having a chance to resist.

The cordial, therefore, is always poured-in subtly and without consent. The victim always has to deal with something that has already happened, only then potentially employing protective aggression in an effort to chase out the intruder. However, even a single drop of the toxic solution changes the colour of the relationship and can no longer be unmixed in order to restore it to the way it was experienced beforehand. This makes aggressively rejecting the intruder very complicated for two main reasons. The first, the clearly aversive experience is hardly ever the first. It is usually preceded by a few cordial drops that were easy not to reject and went in without resistance.

As a result, the victim might feel that he or she had already given up the right to aggressively refuse by not rejecting previous intrusions. My patient, for example, felt that watching pornography with his cousin had already made him an accomplice, which made him unable to reject the activities that followed. Each activity, another cordial drop, made the escalation to follow less likely to be resisted.

The second reason relates to the idea that the cordial drops cannot be unmixed, reversing the relationship to how it was before. As a result, rejecting the intrusion is often experienced as risking this relationship and many others, similar to making a disclosure. My patient recalled how aged 8, as grooming was constantly escalating, he felt that in order to tell his parents about something that he did not want to do with his cousin he would need to confess for all the things he felt that he "agreed to".

For these reasons, protective aggression and with it, the accessibility to actual protective objects and real parents, are often experienced as unavailable as the grooming relational hack takes over. Consequently, anxiety, extreme discomfort, and emotional pain increase and with them the need to find a survivable solution that reduces the pain in the absence of protective aggression.

The grooming experience itself offers a potential solution; as the colour of the cordial only gradually changes, it leaves much room for denial and delusion – imagining the new colour as the original or just a new shade, as a way of surviving the relationship without being able to resist.

To summarise, grooming hacks into internal and external relational structures, rendering protective aggression ineffective. Essentially, the hack disconnects aggression from a sense of a good benevolent internal object providing safety and potency. In addition, it disconnects it from the idea that it can be safely discharged, experienced, and tolerated. Many of these loose disconnected aggression-related relational threads are then unconsciously misconnected. Identifying with the abuser, for example, might be a misconnection of aggression to a bad object. An omnipotent passive victim position might be a misconnection of aggression to passivity, creating the familiar picture in which a sense of mastery over the abuse is achieved by numbness and repetition, or oscillations between feeling powerless and finding refuge in addiction, obsessive revenge fantasies, chronic resentments, impotent bouts of rage, or dreams of magic success and getting away.

The victim's perspective of grooming

As I have already mentioned, grooming usually starts with a first minor incident which already includes the ingredients of the escalation to follow. Those ingredients form the first few drops of the toxic cordial described by my patient; there is a small request to do something against one's actual wishes, beliefs, and feelings. The request usually takes the victim by surprise so that he finds himself involved in something before noticing or being able to think about what is going on.

This first experience is already extremely harmful because it is the moment the perpetrator places a foot at the victim's door. The next time another aversive experience knocks, the capacity to shut the door would be further reduced. Many patients expressed versions of the following quote, "Once I didn't reject the first act, I felt that I could not say no to the next thing". Interestingly, all of them described similar experiences of passivity in which they never say yes but do not experience themselves as effectively resisting either. Their passivity and lack of resistance are then actively misinterpreted by the perpetrator as "consent". Many victims often perceive their experience in the same way, unable to take into account the inherent power difference between victim and perpetrator, feeling that they could and even should have resisted and not doing so was a sign of collusion and weakness.

The foot at the door grooming process hacks into the victim, steals the authority to say no, and leaves a corrupt presence behind, an invisible code that prevents the door from ever being locked again.

This process is very similar to what Christopher Bolas (1987) describes as *extractive introjection* – a violent intersubjective theft of an emotional experience, mental structure, or idea in which the perpetrator robs the victim of the freedom to have an independent, separate experience. Bolas suggests that the theft results in the victim feeling "… surprise, shock, acute anxiety and fear, humiliation, concealment and dread", experiences all grooming victims recollect on their journey of trying to reclaim the stolen aspects of their experiences.

I believe that this is the essence of sexual exploitation – the breaking in and the corruption of one of the most important psychological structures – the ability to use aggression to protect the self. Once the entry code had been stolen and changed, the victim is depleted of the power to resist now and in the future, needing to survive by other psychological means.

Corruption, the secret code left behind by the exploiting hacker, is central to grooming and the establishment of an abusive internal culture. It creates a situation in which the passive resistant part of the personality is no longer protected by its passivity because it becomes an observer of abuse.

The relationship between this passive observer and the part of the personality participating in the abuse is central to understanding the narrative and culture of each abusive relationship.

One common psychic solution is the creation of a split between the body and the mind; the body is perceived as either detached and frozen or actively engaged in the abuse. The mind is perceived as either trapped and suffering or dissociated, as in an "out of body experience".

In fact, as in most of the cases of grooming and abuse I have come across, the actual experience is a mixture of detachment, dissociation, and participation, leading to intense confusion in perceiving the reality of what is going on. In treatment, patients often come in contact with this confusion for the first time and start disentangling the various threads of their actual experiences, the meanings they attributed to them at the time, and their new reflections in therapy. A Patient once reflected on his experience of treatment and said, "at the beginning of therapy I thought the abuse was all my fault and I hated myself. Then I realised that I was a victim, which put some order in my mind but made me feel vulnerable and furious ... moving on from that victim position was the hardest thing; this is when therapy really started".

What this patient meant was that although realising he was a victim helped disentangle some of his experience, it was only a first stage in noticing the reality of what had happened. The therapy that followed was the process in which the structural damages of the grooming process had to be noticed and attended to. This specific patient noticed how he repeatedly perverted his aggression by either victimising himself (consenting to sex he did not actually want) or excitedly participating in the humiliation of others, which dominated his masturbation fantasies. Again and again, he described the same experience; his conscious mind only becoming alert to the emotional reality of what was going on "too late" when things started to happen or just as they ended. The patient moved from describing his destructive behaviours as something he "had to get rid of" to something he was addicted to and struggled "to let go of". Successful treatment depended on the development (or restoration) of good protective aggression – the system before the grooming hack was introduced or an alternative un-hacked totally new protective culture. The patient then experienced a sense of choice; he could go with the "hacked into system" and slip into the familiar cycle, or tolerate the risk inherent to making a stand, and resist.

Clinical examples

Gary (now 23) is an example of almost complete participation. He remembered a moment of total emersion in the abuse (aged 9) when he surprised his abuser with a sexual act the abuser did not expect, something Gary learned from the pornography he watched rather than from the abuser himself. In hindsight, Gary talked about "taking the initiative" as the moment he stopped being a victim and took the abuse as a dare that he had to enact. In his state of total emersion, Gary did not only identify with the abuser's aims but triumphed over them and the abuser, leaving the experience of being overwhelmed, hurt and powerless far behind him. Indeed, although Gary remembered his abuse in detail, he only realised he was abused years after this contact ended. His participation and emersion were so deep that he totally dissociated from his experience as a victim and distorted the meaning of his experience.

Gary's total participation depended on the quality of the grooming process and the way he survived it by identifying with the corruption of the resistant, passive, observing part of the personality. As I have explained before, the grooming hacker leaves a corrupt code behind to replace the stolen authority to resist. It "bribes" the resistant-passive observer with a promise of omnipotence – a key to triumphing over the whole experience by becoming even more powerful than the abuser. From feeling oppressed and victimised the observer turns from passivity into action by becoming an internal "cult leader", daring himself to outmanoeuvre the abuser and triumph over him by taking the lead.

Donna (16) was referred as a consultation case to her residential children's home. I chose to describe her case here because of the impact her behaviour had on her environment and the way this represented the core of her experience and difficulties.

The history of the case was very scarce apart for one significant report; when Dona was about eight, she saw her father being violent to her mother and then saw them having sexual intercourse. This was not reported by Donna but by an older cousin who was there with her at the time. A social services investigation resulted in the father leaving the family home after further disclosures of a long history of violence between the parents. Donna had very little contact with her father since.

In primary school, Donna presented as very bright and academically able. She spent many hours studying and reading for her pleasure. Apart for the one traumatic memory reported, which she also remembered, she stated that she could not recall anything else, neither traumatic nor pleasurable. Transferring to secondary school was described as easy because Donna was accepted to a good school based on her academic achievements. She initially did very well, as though in denial of any transitions. However, maybe because Donna was very beautiful and attractive, her efforts at denial and hiding were countered by constant challenges from her peers. She noticed how boys became interested in her and she began to perceive other girls as competitive. At that point, aged fourteen, her behaviour deteriorated very rapidly. Aged 15, she was no longer interested in school and spent her time with gang-affiliated boys who were into drugs and criminality. Her mother was exasperated, worried, and outraged by her behaviour. Donna ran away from home a few times and was found with known gang members. She was rumoured to be the girlfriend of a much older gang leader and presented as dismissive and contemptuous of the adults who attempted to set boundaries and engage her constructively. She was placed in a residential care home following a violent attack on another girl from the educational unit she now attended. The girl called her a whore and in response Donna drew a blade and cut her, causing injuries that required stitches on the victim's arms and hands. A police and social services investigation produced a narrative of severe exploitation;

Donna was passed between gang members for sex and was used to traffic drugs to different parts of the country. Professionals were extremely concerned and described Donna as a very vulnerable young person.

In consulting to the residential unit she now lived in, it became clear that Donna perceived herself as neither vulnerable nor exploited. In fact, as in many other cases, those were the two experiences she was psychologically focused on avoiding and projecting into others through her extreme behaviours. The staff looking after her found it extremely difficult to do so. They were overtly negative, often scared and feeling victimised by her actions. In response, they were either placatory, trying to have an easy shift, or punitive and over controlling, avoiding feeling powerless and humiliated through action.

Although Donna was clearly exploited, she felt powerful. She was triumphant in being chosen for sex by the powerful gang leader and in her capacity to then use her body to provide sex as part of her gang-role. The close link between that and the aggressive "protection" provided by the male-violent gang, the money and the drugs, became a very omnipotent and addictive serum. The attempts by professionals to address Donna as a victim or try to help her notice her vulnerability were experienced by her as assaults – purposeful efforts to make her weak and unprotected. She responded, like many others, with violence and absconding, projecting vulnerability, victimisation, and rage into those who attempted to help her.

David (18) was referred after disclosing an addiction to violent and disturbing pornography. In the assessment, he disclosed years of childhood sexual abuse by an older brother. In therapy, he slowly became able to describe the various aspects of that experience; Unlike Gary and Donna, David talked about hating his brother from the very beginning of the abuse. He never wanted to do what his brother wanted but "either said nothing or OK, never yes or no", leaving him feeling that he has repeatedly failed to protect himself. "Taking part", as he experienced it at the time, made it difficult to tell his parents about it. He felt guilty and ashamed and wanted to protect them from the knowledge of what was happening to him. Psychologically, the split between participation and resistance was enacted as a split between David's mind and body. The body was participating, immersed, excited, and dissociated from the mind that was holding on to the resistance and psychological pain. The internal corrupt code left by the hacking perpetrator seemed to repeatedly overpower the resistant observer by inhibiting aggression and going straight to the participating body.

David described a memory that helped understand this dynamic; He was with his brother in their usual hideout. He was very distressed and saying that he did not want to do it again, begging his brother to stop. In response, the brother became pseudo kind and persuasive. On one hand, he told David that they did not have to do anything if David did not want to. On the other hand, if David agreed, they could do something, not David pleasuring his brother but the brother pleasuring David. Similar to many other boys who had been abused in this way, David talked about the terrible difficulty to say no at this point, as the abuser was gently gaining access to his body and he watched with horror how the body seemed to welcome this with physical excitement whilst his mind froze, stifling both fear and intense aggression. David's body was hacked into, bypassing his mind. It was another evidence of the corruption induced by grooming, the presence of the hacker's internal agent that could open the door from within and allow the abuser in.

The young people presented here are examples to the ways the personality survives abuse without the protection of benign aggression. It functions in a variety of ways and combinations with the aim of minimising pain and surviving moment to moment. As presented in the clinical examples, this is always a highly destructive process that can present as very internal and secretive, external and challenging, or a mixture of both.

The perpetrator's perspective of grooming

Henry, an adolescent patient who described how he perfected a system of seducing young boys to send him naked pictures of themselves, talked about being able to tell if an initial *no* had the potential to be converted into something else. He said, "I am the master of removing a NO and placing an OK instead". For Henry, the picture was only a trophy to his capacity to get in and perform the theft. Indeed, his sexuality was not even paedophilic. He sexualised the grooming process and got excited by the moment of triumph at the end of it – the picture – the evidence of his power to get someone to do something they did not want to do and was harmful to them, behind the back of parents.

Some of the victim–perpetrator dynamics that I have encountered was further confused by the fact that it might have been the perpetrator's first experience in crossing this boundary. Here, the pace of grooming was not as calculated and rehearsed compared to that of an experienced offender. Instead, the perpetrator presented as conflicted and disorganised. One abuser I have worked with said that he felt very guilty but was unable to make himself stop. Instead, he expected the victim to resist and got very worried when this did not happen. Obviously, at the time, he was not conscious of already disabling the victim's authority to object by being the victim's trusted older friend. All harmful intentions towards the victim remained mostly unconscious until they were actually enacted. There was an internal split between the conscious part of the perpetrator that did not want to hurt the victim to an unconscious part of him that groomed the victim to accept further escalations.

Similar to the victim, who no longer had the capacity to say no, this particular perpetrator experienced an inability to object to his own actions and stop. He then projected this internal dynamic into the victim by stealing the victim's capacity to object on one hand and desperately wishing that the victim would stop him on the other. Luckily, this perpetrator eventually got so scared and ashamed of his intentions that he acted out in a way that caused him to get noticed and be stopped.

Other perpetrators are more callous and organised. Indeed, all perpetrators have a first time too. Getting caught after the first time, especially for an adolescent or even a young adult, is a sign of hope because it means that the perpetrator had allowed something to leak out (either consciously or unconsciously), had not perfected the grooming process, and effectively delegated the need to be stopped to the environment. It is an invitation for a benign external authority to step in, use protective aggression, say stop, and set the world straight by using its authority and power in a benevolent way.

Not being caught, on the other hand, keeps the abuse secret, fosters omnipotence, and prevents any external authority from stopping harm from occurring. The benign sense of protective aggression is then corrupted by the hacking grooming perpetrator to the point of being totally unavailable to the victim or even further perverted and distorted.

From a perpetrator's point of view, the abuse, like any enactment, is a perverse solution to unresolved internal conflicts. Without getting into a discussion about the perverse act itself, it is important to keep in mind that it is the product of distortion of reality and of the truth (McDougall, 1972; Chasseguet-Smirguel, 1981, 1985; Steiner, 1993). The actual dynamic of grooming, the theft of the capacity to resist and the corruption positioned in its place, is an example of how this distortion is operationalised, becomes relational, and prescribed to the victim, who then takes it on as some kind of an "alternative truth" about themselves.

The perpetrator psychologically depends on this abusive solution, which can then, when enacted, become highly addictive. By becoming the substance of this addiction, the victim is forced to accommodate the abuser's perverse structure in which reality and truth are denied and perverted.

Donna, the girl I presented earlier, spent her childhood observing her parents' confusing relationship, a mix of ordinariness, violence, coercion, control, and sex. A sense of a benign protective aggression was never available for her to experience. Instead, she seemed to have internalised a perverse concoction that paved the way to future hackers and exploiters.

As an example, it is important to acknowledge in this context a common phenomenon, best described by a patient that used to be violent to his wife. He said, "if a man slaps a woman in the street, it is very unlikely that they would then go home together unless they are married". Outside the realm of an abusive relationship, hurting someone else would usually result in a fight or the victim running away. Hurting the groomed victim within a slowly developing abusive relationship, on the other hand, means that he or she had lost their ability to protect themselves and therefore cannot leave.

Recovering protective aggression

In my work with victims and perpetrators of abuse, I have noticed that understanding and insight are not enough to propel meaningful change. They are necessary to evoke the wish to change and the need to develop protective aggression, but without taking action in the real world, many patients remain stuck ruminating about a potent future but trapped in cycles of addiction or sadomasochism in which they commit to moving on and then watch themselves destroying this potential.

Heather Wood (2013) discusses perversion and psychological addiction and argues that patients do not change by developing insight alone. They only start showing signs of recovery after they use the insight in order to come in real contact with the traumas at the core of the defensive, perverse, addictive structures.

Those trying to recover from the psychological devastation in the aftermath of grooming and abuse are often similar to the patients described by Wood. However, I think that even coming in contact with the actual trauma might not be enough sometimes. Noticing the criminal act of grooming and abuse and rightfully assigning blame to the perpetrator is not enough either. As I have mentioned before, my patients only start to recover when they begin to develop or re-own their aggression and work through their relationship to authority.

The therapeutic process, therefore, attempts to repair the damage done by the theft of the victim's authority to resist and the replacement of it with a corrupt internal code that entangles the victim with the perpetrator's addictive perverse needs.

Recovering from being exploited is, therefore, much more that repairing an experience of being hurt. It requires a reconstruction of authenticity, separating lies from the truth, pain from pleasure, and, at times, restoring lost elements of the natural facts of life such as generational differences, the need for protection, being part of a family or a group. Restoring these basics then allows for the establishment of a good sense of agency and aggression, which replaces collusion, rage, humiliation, and revenge fantasies. Feeling protected, the self no longer depends on the methods developed to survive the abuse without the capacity to resist it.

Treatment

It is important to state here that the patients I work with are those who continue to cope with their past abusive experiences by maintaining an internal corrupt culture. They enact this internal structure through a variety of destructive behaviours, some of which are very addictive, some perverse, violent, or harmful to others.

Their internal structure and the way it is enacted have a direct impact on the therapeutic relationship. I find it impossible to relate to these patients without being groomed into accommodating the patient's unconscious invitation to join the passive-observer part of his personality. As a result, I often arrive at an impasse, passively watching how my patients use the sessions well on the one hand, able to experience insight and make real contact, but on the other hand, act out, as if forcing me to helplessly watch their destructive activity, attack, and perversion of the therapeutic work. Together with the patient, I become an expert in understanding what went wrong and how things continue to be destructive and perverted, unable to become proficient in making things right again.

This often presents a clinical dilemma which can be addressed on a few levels simultaneously. First of all, it is important to acknowledge how the therapist has become entangled in the patient's passivity and enactment, only able to watch without acting to resist and stop the patient from hurting themselves or others.

Although the interpretation does not change the overall structure, which remains destructive, it helps develop a sense of some internal freedom to think. This freedom, however, is not equal to an authority to act, which carries with it further risks. As a result, although patients begin to think freely inside sessions, they still act to attack this freedom outside the session's setting. It is as if the patient in the room – the victim, fills the session with complaining about the patient outside the room – the perpetrator, the addict, the self-harmer, the one who acts to destroy the therapist's or group's work. Indeed, many of these destructive activities occur on the night before the session or even on the way to the clinic in order to provide an experience of being in the aftermath of something destructive, something the group or psychotherapist can no longer prevent.

Anyone working therapeutically or looking after young people presenting in this way is likely to be embroiled in these addictive cycles. Becoming part of the cycle and therefore responding as if reading from a script written and directed by the patients' unconscious leads to an impasse. However, if one remains completely outside of the cycle, one will probably wait forever for the patient to join and step out of the script whilst never helping the patient develop the capacity and authority to do so.

The possible solution to this, I believe, lies in the psychotherapist's general stance, which depends mainly on his or her actual belief in their patient's right and capacity to get better. As Ann Alvarez (2012) argues, psychotherapists sometimes need to hold on to the patients' sense of hope when this is not available to them. Groups act in this way quite instinctively sometimes, whilst individual psychotherapists might struggle with the concept because it requires taking an active stance towards the patient and changing the interpretative style. Following Alvarez (2012), I often interpret protective aggression as "currently unavailable" rather than lacking or absent, creating a potential for hope rather than join the patient's despair or perverse excitement.

I usually become conscious of my entanglement when I don't completely believe in what I say to patients: Although the interpretations seem to have the correct content, they never sound or feel right. Instead, they become part of a defensive psychological manoeuvre designed to give me the illusion of being able to think freely without clearly addressing my actual position in relation to the patient. As I suggested before, I become an expert in predicting the patient's behaviour and how things go wrong, which they usually do. I lose any real hope or imagination of how things can get better and the responsibility I have to helping my patient achieve that.

The following example might clarify this point; A 15-year-old young man, with traumatic early life experiences, was referred following a conviction of the attempted rape of a young woman. He initially presented as respectful and interested in thinking to such an extent that it was impossible to imagine that the young man sitting with me was the same young man who almost raped a woman in the park. At some point towards the end of an extended assessment, he spoke about a particular funny YouTube clip that he had seen. Casually addressing me in the session, he said that he would like to show me the clip on his phone. I refused, saying that it would be better if he could just tell me about it. He seemed not to notice what I said and proceeded to take his phone out of his pocket. I stayed silent, holding on to the initial comment I had just made. My internal discourse at that point sounded like "let's see what he does with it …". The patient got up, walked to my chair, pressed play, and shoved the phone right in front of my eyes. Before I had a chance to refuse again, which I actively did by standing up, I had already seen something of what he wanted me to see.

As I have said before, these are naturally occurring experiences with these patients, both victims and perpetrators, often leading to some enactment in the consulting room, which is actually helpful in understanding the dynamic. Indeed, it became very clear to me at that point that this young man was a perpetrator – he was not only "not taking no for an answer" but eradicating the no altogether.

Apart from the obvious experience of a boundary being crossed, it was important for me to notice how my interpretation represented my wish to be understood by the patient, who would then stop doing what he was doing rather than presenting him with active and assertive resistance. In fact, the interpretation was a *no* already eager to occupy a passive observer's position rather than a refusal said with an intention to be respected. As mentioned above, I was unaware at the moment that I was already being hacked into and acting to survive this moment of violation rather than use my protective aggression by assertively resisting it.

This experience is also common in work with severely traumatised and abused children who are violent and highly dis-regulated. Therapists and other professionals often find themselves in a position in which they feel that they are either their patient's victims, "accepting" bullying and violence as experiences to be tolerated, or, on the other hand, become preoccupied with "consequences" to bad behaviour, taking action to over-control and limit those they are caring for. In the consulting room, we might make all the right interpretations about a child's emotional states whilst simultaneously avoid acting in a way that expresses benign authority. Like victims, we expect our violent patients to understand our interpretations and then stop hurting us, or when occupying the controlling punitive position, we strongly feel that a child needs to be disciplined rather than offered treatment as if the experience of having real authority and providing psychotherapy were mutually exclusive. As a result, authority is either fantasised or harsh, not active and benevolent, corresponding to patients' traumatic experiences of being hacked-into and their protective aggression disabled and perverted.

Authority and leadership are often absent from the discourse of individual psychotherapy and kept only within the discipline of group relations. Similarly, aggression as a capacity is often forgotten, especially when thinking about it as an integral part of a therapeutic intervention. Yet, when working with children and young people, the psychotherapist is the only adult in the room, the one who sets the rules of the setting, starts and stops sessions. Those are always acts that must include benign aggression and are, therefore, often challenged in a variety of ways.

The direction therapy takes over time is usually towards disentangling the various experiential aspects of the trauma by inspecting its ingredients as expressed through enactments and the therapeutic relationship. My general experience is that clarity of reflection usually exposes the corruption at the core of the organisation and the main agent inhibiting and perverting aggression.

When patients begin to experience potent aggression for the first time, by being assertive, for example, they quickly notice how the impulse to act out destructively is markedly reduced. Patients typically describe how being firm meant that they could put a conflict behind them rather than spend a long time ruminating on humiliation and revenge.

A young man who spent many years in treatment has recently noticed how he no longer actually experiences his old triggers for enactment. He does not feel compelled to think about his past abuse, he is no longer intruded by memories, and he does not feel anxious that he is a potential predator as before. However, he is still engaged with his old destructive behaviour, now with open eyes, feeling that he needs to invest a lot of effort in order to be self-destructive because it is no longer his second nature. In one significant session, he said that in the past, he felt that he was worthy of his self-abuse because he felt he was a pervert. Now, when he is being destructive, it felt as if he was "hurting an innocent man". Hurting an innocent man – his self – was now masochistic rather than the reactive addictive cycle of the past. Standing up and protecting the innocent internal victim required aggression, which was corrupted by grooming and unavailable at the time of the abuse. The patient was actually experiencing the availability of the aggression he needed to stop the abuse in his mind but perverted it because he was too scared of making a commitment to a life without all his old solutions to psychological pain.

David, the patient presented earlier, had been in therapy for more than five years. In this time, he oscillated between passivity and resistance until he became able to resist most of his addictive destructive behaviours. His position of recovery lasted about two years. David experienced a sense of authority and growth during this time in many aspects of his life. However, his sessions were completely emptied out of meaning, as if the only thing David could do was declare that he was no longer harming himself. As a result, David hardly spoke.

David's capacity to avoid harm was, in fact, an act of false generosity (Freire, 1970), a kind of a charitable option provided to him by his internal abusive regime in exchange for not aggressively rejecting it. He was granted a sense of false freedom, a walk in the prison yard, in order not to face his fear of what real resistance might entail. Being in this recovery position has hindered his overall capacity to use aggression. He has struck a deal with the internal corrupt hacked into structure.

In order to regain a fighting spirit and lead a new resistance, David first had to relapse into a dangerous state of enactments. However, he was no longer silent in his sessions. He described the level of his self-destruction in full detail and for the first time. He linked it to new revelations regarding his past experiences, mainly to memories of being groomed before the abuse, feeling that then he could have still resisted but had been unable to.

Ending

Ending treatment with these patients hardly ever feels as a complete piece of work because not many patients leave feeling that they can completely refrain from self-destructive behaviour or other disturbance. As described above, some patients might become highly perverse in relation to themselves and their psychotherapy as a way of imposing an impasse and negating ending and separateness. Other patients stop their destructive behaviours at a price of inhibiting their overall activities, as if "suspending life". They too, are unable to use aggression constructively and attempt to avoid it altogether in order not to pervert it.

Reviewing a few patients at six months and a year following the end of treatment revealed a very significant piece of work that they did on their own. Only following the ending could they fully own a sense of authority and act on it without the temptation to corrupt the process in order to control the therapist and delay the end of the therapeutic relationship. On their own, knowing and accepting the separation from their therapist or group, the last phase of development could take place.

References

Alvarez, A. (2012) *The Thinking Heart*, Oxford: Routledge.

Bolas, C. (1987) *The Shadow of the Object*, London: Free Association Books.

Chasseguet-Smirguel (1985) *The ego ideal: A psychoanalytic essay on the Malady of the Ideal*, London: Free Association Books.

Freire, P. (1970) *Pedagogy of the Oppressed*, New York: Harder and Harder.

Freud, A. (1972) *The Child as a Person in His Own Right, The Psychoanalytic Study of the Child*. https://doi.org/10.1080/00797308.1972.11822730

McDougall, J (1972) Primal scene and sexual perversion. *The International Journal of Psychoanalysis, 53*(3), 371–384.

Steiner, J (1993) *Psychic Retreats. Pathological Organizations in Psychotic, Neurotic and Borderline Patients*, London: Tayor and Francis.

Wood, H. (2013) 'The nature of the addiction in "sex addiction" and paraphilias', in Bower, M., Hale, R. and Wood, H. (eds) *Addictive States of Mind*, London: Karnac.

5

VICTIM/VICTIMIZER

Grappling with some of the dynamics of exploitation

Robin Solomon

On the face of it, if someone is a victim then logically, there must be a victimizer. To be abused one needs an abuser. The 'done to' needs a 'do-er'. Suggesting that there is something more complex and nuanced than these binary positions is not the same as blaming the victims. Someone can be a 'participant' and still be a victim – often of intergenerational or early developmental trauma or impacted upon by deficits in social or familial roles or experiences both external and internal. These deficits impinge on the development of trust in the early containing environment, and adversely affect the establishment of the internal templates of self and others. These templates form the backdrop of vulnerability to exploiting relationships.

It is the unconscious, unknown or un-reflected upon aspects of these internal dynamics that make them so difficult to work with. It can feel like the young person does not want it to be different. Child Sexual Exploitation is distinct from other types of assault or rape, where physical strength, threats of violence, or the abrogation of generational boundaries are specific defining features. Incest and early years sexual abuse are a subsection of the latter but can also sow the seeds for the former.

It is reassuring that the social and political domains of child sexual exploitation and child criminal exploitation are finally being examined more forensically and through increasing research, yet the psychological domain has been less remarked upon. In this chapter, I hope to suggest a few concepts drawn from psychoanalytic perspectives that might help frontline workers have more efficacy.

In the aftermath of the Rochdale and Rotherham investigations into child sexual exploitation, there was a great deal of reportage, and I listened with great interest to the interviews with some of the young people, mostly females,

DOI: 10.4324/9781003020370-5

mostly in state care. In one television documentary, the interviewer, a sensitive journalist, asked a young woman how many times she had met the men who had abused her. She thought for a moment and replied something to the effect of, 'forty? fifty? – dunno'. The journalist, sympathising with the young woman, went on to say that this young woman hadn't known she was a victim until her social worker told her. The idea of 'victimhood' is a helpful but insufficient label that can often become a block to further understanding or therapeutic intervention. The term 'victim' potentially becomes a label that offers a social narrative but one that only partially explains the confusing internal experience.

As in the case of Ghislaine Maxwell, unusually a female predator, she appeared blind to how her own early childhood experiences had impacted on her becoming an active participant alongside Jeffrey Epstein in the exploitation of other young women. The complex debate about her own victimhood only came to be spotlighted in the media as a significant aspect of her defence and sentencing. The media coverage became quite polarised – was she a guilty victimizer or a blameless victim? The coverage of Maxwell and other high-profile cases also brought into the debate a complex area – how could the victim become a victimizer? This is often an area of confusion prison officers can face in young offenders' institutions – do they punish the perpetrator or treat them as the victim of abuse at an earlier stage?

When victims become exploiters?

During a consultation with a social worker, she told me about JR, a 14-year-old young woman in local authority care. The social worker felt she had been working hard over a number of months to establish a relationship with this rejecting and demanding young person who was described as a 'victim of early abuse and neglect at home, exposure to domestic violence, and with the likelihood of intra-familial sexual abuse'. Given her over sexualised presentation and indiscriminate relationships, all the professionals were concerned about the possibility of sexual exploitation.

She was placed with very experienced foster carers. Despite 'agreeing' to the house rules, she started to leave the house not saying where she was going, and come back much later than the agreed return, and often with gifts or money that she refused to discuss. Drunk and argumentative, there would often be bruising around her throat and thighs. After a period of time, some of this behaviour diminished and the carers, the mental health practitioner, social workers and school outreach professionals all started to feel things were improving. When to the network's surprise, this 'more settled' JR was arrested by the police for extorting money from a vulnerable adult male through threats of violence towards his family. Texts uncovered by the police revealed her offering this young adult man the potential of sexual relations, escalating to threats of exposing his sexual interest and then to violence if money was not given to her.

Instead, his family went to the police and she was arrested. On being released to the care of the social worker who was at the police station with her, pending further investigation, JR smiled and said, 'they can't charge me; I'm a looked after young person; I'm a victim'. The social worker, said she felt angry, but on reflection was not sure whom she was angry with. This confusion made her feel uncertain about what to do and left her feeling guilty. The victim-perpetrator paradigm (Jankowitz 2018) describes a phenomenon in which groups rely on exclusive constructions of victimhood to support their favourable self-image and emphasise the differentiation between themselves and groups they label as perpetrators. Certainly, JR would not identify herself as an exploiter.

But how does the exploited JR become the exploiting JR, or find herself in other relationships that continue to exploit her despite the determined efforts of the professional adults around her. It is these lesser explored/ unconscious aspects of these invidious relationships rather than solely the social context, important as that is, that continue to leave the young person vulnerable and difficult to engage in work that provides opportunities for development and change.

When there is a media scandal, the public find it impossible to understand how these young victims were not kept safe. The network of professionals, residential staff, social workers, the police and schools are often blamed. The idea that in some investigations into the scandals, there were some who called it a 'lifestyle choice' seemed incomprehensible. Yet to those adults without a way to understand this participation as a result of earlier victimisation, they felt frustrated and angry when all of their attempts at nurture and care were rejected and rebuffed and they felt out of control or inadequate for not being able to change the behaviours or keep the young people safe. To them, it felt like the young person had made a choice. Exploited young people cannot be in touch with their own feelings of powerlessness or shame. Instead, these can be unconsciously pushed away and into others who come to experience those feelings as their own.

In my work consulting to residential staff teams and individual practitioners dealing with some of the most vulnerable and exploited young people, one of the ideas that they have found helpful is that of 'repetition compulsion' a term coined by Freud in 1914 but still useful today because it attempts to explain how people continue to be drawn to others in new relationships in ways which replicate the internal self and other from their earliest experiences. This includes recreating the relationship and event or putting oneself in situations that have a high probability of it occurring again. Freud suggested that there are two ways people manage their trauma; either processing it and turning it into a painful but working memory or re-enacting it again and again in a concrete way Freud (1914).

This compulsion to recreate unconsciously the abuse and exploitation of earlier years might help to explain how these young people's response to the adults who tried to stop them – saying that 'they wanted' to see these men, or that they 'had a right to meet whoever they wanted, and that staff couldn't stop them' – was so confusing and felt like a purposeful choice. For some of these young women, when approached by the groomers and predators who search them out, and part of the groomers' psyche is its ability to identify groups of young people whose situation is characterised by their vulnerability, this connection becomes almost magnetic. There is more of a pull towards an unconscious familiarity with something in these perpetrators and the physical contact that they offer than to the unfamiliar unconscious scripts of caring, helpful, curious and reflective professionals.

It is not to say that the external realities of money, gifts, or other consumer goods are not part of what draws those in poverty, deprivation, despair or depression to get enticed into these trafficking gangs, be drawn to sexual predators or stay with the groomers. But it is not a sufficient explanation, nor can it explain those in more privileged situations being drawn in. To understand it, one may have to consider an idea of a compulsion to recreate earlier relational templates. In those early relationships, there had been no satisfactory or appropriately available adult to help process frightening and abusive experiences. Therapeutic interventions often consist of trying to think about how the early trauma relates to the current situation. Putting these pieces together is painful and frightening. These are young people who run from those who try to help them think.

In repetition compulsion, we keep recreating these situations and relationships because we repressed them or haven't processed them. According to Stubley (2023), we return to them in the hope that it will be different. For these young people who have experienced abuse or neglect, it is often the inexpressible wish that they could get the parents or family they hoped they would have rather than the one they did. But this is what is so hard to face. So advice or sympathy alone, however well intended, does not resolve this. To develop, one has to grieve the loss of the good experience, to grieve for what was not available or what you can't have. Without that, this grief can get stuck as grievance and prevent using the availability of others or even experiencing others as the focus of your grievance.

Another curious dynamic of child sexual exploitation is how the victim becomes the victimizer and the complex dynamics that tie the abuser and abused together. This might be thought about as having the quality of sadomasochism. This is particularly relevant in working with adolescents. Betty Joseph (1982) noted that in this stage of development, there is a tendency for adolescents who are troubled to turn to destructive or self-destructive behaviour. Those who are exploited may display suicidal ideation, self-harm, self-starvation and inappropriate sexual behaviour. This can be profoundly shocking and alarming to others, especially if the young person seems to enjoy the impact it has on others. Joseph describes these young people as gaining pleasure both by harming himself and the helping relationship. Understanding this dynamic is important for anyone who works with this population. Of course, not all destructive and self-destructive behaviours come into that category. Glasser (1979) identified what he saw as the difference between aggression and sadism as being located in the attitude to the other. In the aggressive act, the destruction and negation of the other is a core feature. In the sadistic act, the emotional reaction of the other is crucial and the aim is to cause the other to suffer. A useful thing to keep in mind when working with these young people is the possibility that unconsciously the young person needs to make the helper suffer or to be provoked into causing the young person to feel suffering.

Joseph (1982) described the development of an internal situation dominated by these dynamics as beginning in childhood when the child experiences pain that can intensify into torment. The child becomes identified with the internalised tormentor and inflicts pain on herself. But the crucial factor in this phenomenon is that the pain becomes perversely exciting. It can be that this excitement, a manic rush away from thinking, which becomes almost like an addiction.

One example of this was a young woman who had been moved from an inpatient hospital unit to a residential home. She had repetitive episodes of going to her bedroom, sitting on the bed and banging her head on the wall. This could go on and on. The staff spent hours with her, shielding her head, padding the wall with pillows and restraining her. They felt worried and distressed and, on several occasions, had to call for an ambulance. Staff noted it had a mindless quality about it; one said it was as if she was 'knocking out her own brain'. Yet she seemed to enjoy the drama that unfolded around her and screamed that they were hurting her when they tried to intervene.

A problem for staff working in close proximity to such young people is that they may experience the young person as the tormentor. Without a framework for thinking about these processes and helpful reflective supervision, there could also be the possibility that workers' own ghosts can become activated unknowingly and elicit their own more provoking qualities. These might manifest as inappropriate teasing or nagging in the guise of humour or persisting in a plan that is not working. A residential care worker recently told me how a young person laughed and threw a plate at her 'for no reason', saying all she'd been doing was joking with her to get her to do something. For the young person, the persistent chivvying her to do something had felt tormenting until she retaliated concretely – throwing something that hurt and thinking it was funny.

Joining a gang

In the same way, a further counter-intuitive aspect of understanding sexual exploitation is often the intense bonds which can exist between victims and exploiters. It is hard to understand why the young people 'join' the gang.

Gang mentality exists in families, in criminality and in street life, but there are also gangs in the mind. Both Canham (2002) and Cregeen (2008) draw on the work of Rosenfeld to explore how these states of mind take hold when working with adolescents in residential settings. Group and gang states of mind may be perceived as present within individuals and within groups, and they reflect and produce dynamics intra-psychically and inter-psychically. Canham describes how when the more positive attributes of group life are prominent, for example, a well-functioning staff team or the young residents enjoying a holiday together or discussing house rules in a residents' meeting, there is a possibility of concern for each other. At an individual level, each member preserves his or her own internally integrated identity or sense of self. There remains a capacity to reflect and there is a predominantly benign atmosphere. When this works it provides meaning and pleasure to membership of a group or to an individual's experience of themselves. In some residential homes where all of the residents have had abusive and neglectful early lives and no safe adults, the group like state is hard to achieve and when it happens is often fleeting. By contrast, a gang-like state of mind emerges, and the anxieties and early defences can mirror the anxieties and defences associated with an infant state of mind. Like pre-cognitive infants they communicate through emotional impact rather than processed thinking. A gang mentality therefore is one in which destructive forces have taken over the group. In gang behaviour, the reign of terror is directed towards other groups. A gang is anti-thought, anti-grown ups and anti-life. The leader of the gang works hard to make sure that everybody knows it would be dangerous to leave – a clear projection of his own knowledge that he would be in danger without them (Canham 2002).

For so many being drawn into Sexual Exploitation, early experience may create that 'gang state of mind'. The associated physical, psychological and emotional changes of adolescents can become a trigger for a powerful move away from helpful adults in the way that all adolescents developmentally separate from their parents. But for these adolescents, the earlier ordinary developmental separation of toddlerhood that needs to take place as a foundation for adolescent separation may have been distorted by the dysfunctional parental relationships of their infancy. It goes some way as well in being able to appreciate the barrage of aggression and opposition that residential care staff can face when working with groups of these complex and vulnerable residents. For staff working in these homes, it can feel at times like a 'reign of terror'.

County line drug dealing, or Child Criminal Exploitation, is another form of exploitation. These young people may often have been witness to early relationships of coercive control, an unconscious form of on-going bullying where one partner exerts power over the other through fear. The abuser may use tactics, such as limiting access to money or monitoring communication in this effort, but rewards compliance with real and emotional gifts. The other person joins the dynamic because it feels safer. Like sexual exploitation where it is sexual activity that leads to additional gains, this gain might take the form of material benefits, i.e., gifts, money, alcohol, drugs or a range of goods. For others, the gain might be acceptance in the group or gang. In criminal or sexual exploitation, there may, in time, be threats or coercion to remain involved. This was the case for 14-year-old Ryan.

He was referred to an adolescent unit because the previous foster care placement had broken down after four years. It had been intended as a long-term placement. But the aggression and violence towards the foster carers increased and they were afraid for themselves and their own young family. Ryan had been removed from a family where violence and bullying were common. Although he says he can't remember, he was present when a man who knew his father was stabbed outside their door. A bright young person, he refused to attend school, demeaning its importance and saying he would go to college when he was ready. Driven by the government guidelines on educational outcomes for looked after children and adolescents (DfE Gov.UK 2014, 2018), the goal of the placement prioritised getting Ryan to school. There was little formulation about emotional goals except to 'form better attachments'.

At the outset, he had a bullying manner, testing staff and every time there was a limit set, he became threatening. He had what seemed to be limited empathy and always responded to questions about why he did things by blaming others for having provoked him. It was always another resident or staff member who was at fault by not complying with his demands. After a huge effort by the staff team to be consistent in responses, supporting each other when under threat, remaining available, articulating how his behaviour made others feel, Ryan, began to settle, spending more time with the staff and other residents rather than out of the home. He was bright and funny, and therefore, it was so much more surprising to social workers and residential staff that he continued to refuse to go to school. After almost two years of incremental progress in building helpful relationships, there was talk by the new social worker that he was going to have to be moved to another placement because this home had not managed to get him to school and, therefore, had not met the educational targets set out in his care plan. It seemed difficult for social workers, pressured by diminishing resources and policy compliance, to step outside the forms or argue with the placement officers and think about how learning relies on being able not to know. For Ryan, in his early life, not knowing or not being in control left him vulnerable.

Ryan had slowly begun to take responsibilities for his role in some of his aggressive behaviours (smashing the TV, kicking in a door) and inching towards the possibility of making amends, rather than always allocating cause and blame to others, in a 'you made me do it by making me angry' response. He had begun to develop better relationships with some of the staff, in particular with the manager with whom he had developed an especially warm relationship and he seemed to respond when she expressed disappointment in his behaviour. One characteristic they all noticed was that he started to ask questions rather than know everything already. Occasionally, Ryan was interested in what he might study 'if' he were to go to school. The social worker, his fourth in the two years he lived there, seemed focused only on the goal of getting Ryan to school. He found it hard to engage with Ryan and had through pressure from his managers started to look for alternative placements. Ryan, getting wind of this plan, retreated to disinterest and kept repeating that he wanted to leave and move to semi-independent living. In this limbo, Ryan started spending more time out of the home. The staff noticed a change in him, an increased secretiveness and a reluctance to spend time with the very staff he had begun to develop good relationships with. A few times, he mentioned the name of a past resident that he ran into in the community – they had realised that they had the children's home in common. What Ryan couldn't know was that the other young person's placement there had broken down because of the extreme violence and criminality of his behaviour and the risk he posed in the home and immediate community. Unusually for the young people living at the home, Ryan had no external criminal incidents since the placement began. An incident, being refused his demand for extra pocket money, led to threatening staff and escalated to property damage and the staff starting to complain about how unmanageable he was. I noted during a consultation that I had not heard Ryan discussed for almost a year until suddenly all progress was lost and I invited them to explore what might be going on.

One afternoon, after reporting Ryan missing the previous night, they were notified that he was in police custody for being with a gang that had assaulted someone the previous evening. On checking his room, the staff found class A drugs in amounts suggesting dealing. There had been no indication of his using anything other than cannabis. Of course, the manager, a tough and streetwise mother herself, was required in keeping with legal and professional responsibilities to notify the police and hand in the drugs. She also knew this would mean that when the gang leader/dealer demanded them back from Ryan – whose role it was in the gang to mind them for him by stashing them in his bedroom – and Ryan couldn't produce them he would be in danger and there would be a risk to other residents and the staff because the building would be targeted by the gang The only possible option was to terminate the placement and move Ryan to another placement, likely far from that location – for his safety and for theirs. Yet on a profound emotional level, she was devastated to abandon this young man who had slowly and painfully made significant emotional contact with staff members.

'If I were his parent' she said, when we were speaking privately, 'I would take the damn drugs, find the gang leader, throw the stuff back in his face, and tell him to leave my son alone, and if he didn't, I would kill him!' Of course, she did not mean that literally and she felt embarrassed for having expressed what she thought were unprofessional feelings. But what she was expressing was what Ryan needed and had never had: a parent who would claim him, keep him safe and not relinquish him. She was emotionally reacting to this abused and neglected boy who denied his dependency needs and vulnerability. Her wish, spoke to the purpose of his placement in residential care. To find a way despite his attempts to destroy it of providing the safe and containing care he had never had. For Ryan, having sensed the pending move planned by the social worker, this had reawakened early feelings of abandonment, rejection and fear and had turned him quickly towards an available gang. Tragically, he was present when members of that gang stabbed a man. Instead of moving from residential care to something more independent, Ryan may face a prison sentence.

Thinking about gangs can help to understand Ryan's move from building trust to joining a gang. From inching towards membership in a residential home group he was drawn to the exploitative gang. In the same way as in child sexual exploitation, criminal exploitation pulls a young person from membership in attempts to provide an experience of a more benign group where concern is possible, into the anti-thought anti-parent destructiveness of the gang. These vulnerable young people have already internalised from their earliest experiences, the dynamics of coercive control. Compliance is integral. But perversely, it can get seen as a choice. Ryan could not bear to know his feelings of powerlessness and rejection with echoes from his past. Instead, some staff carried those feelings unknowingly on Ryan's behalf. Unrecognised feelings can get located in others. The feeling in the staff team was divided between those who were glad to see him go and those who like the manager felt hopeless and sad at the inability for the care system to find better ways of managing these extreme young people.

Something particular to sexual rather than criminal exploitation is, of course, the sexual aspect of exploitative relationships. If the primary caregiver in early relationship uses the baby to meet its own needs, it can evoke a fear in the baby, almost like a loss of self. If, at the same time, the caregiver is neglecting the baby's needs, it exacerbates a fear of abandonment. For the baby, there can be no safe closeness. The closeness or intimacy that is desired is also terrifying and can provoke aggressive feelings to defend against this fear. But the aggression pushes away the very person who is desired. When this combination of neglect of the baby's needs and using the baby to meet the carer's needs is also combined with a history of overt and excessive sexual stimulation by the caregiver, these factors may produce a predisposition to sexualise intolerable emotions and may go some way in helping to thinking about what might be mirrored in the dynamics of child sexual exploitation.

Turning a blind eye

Unlike this reflective manager, many staff and social workers can find it difficult to find a containing space in their own mind for some of these frightened and frightening young people. Pressure, stress and anxiety crowd the thinking space necessary to work effectively with this population. The unbearable, unprocessed feelings of these young people do not get owned or understood by them. Instead, they project those feelings into others. Staff can sometimes get drawn into the internal scripts of the young people, unconsciously acting into the role of the bully or unavailable parent of their early life. For many of these young people, certainly for JR and for Ryan, there was a mother who turned a blind eye to the experience of their child exposed to domestic violence, sexual abuse or other forms of ill treatment.

As early as 1893, Freud drew attention to a state of mind that he described as 'blindness of the seeing eye' in which 'one knows and does not know a thing at the same time' (Britton 1994). While complete denial of reality is an indicator of a more psychotic state, Freud was describing a non-psychotic form of denial, later termed *disavowal*. This was developed into the idea that unlike denial, which defends against reality by not knowing about it, disavowal obliterates only the significance of things, not their existence (Basch 1983; Britton 1994; Bower and Solomon 2018).

Of course, professionals knew that these young women were being groomed, sexually exploited, and running to the perpetrators as they denigrated the staff pleas to stay in, and to stay safe. They knew the gifts were not benign, the intoxication not enjoyable. To hold the narrative of 'lifestyle choice' about these young women was to know and not know something at the same time. Disavowal is different from indifference. Rather than immediately condemning workers and allocating blame, understanding this distinction may help change practices.

An example of this is Sylvia, who came to my office with little appearance of the nervousness or anxiety that often accompanies a first appointment. Instead, she sat down, presenting a feeling of taking control of the space. A young woman of 15, referred because her carers were concerned about sexual exploitation, she was wearing a sleeveless vest and a very short skirt, making it almost impossible for me not to notice the extensive display of scars running down both arms and on her upper thighs. She sat down rather dramatically, crossed her legs and bent forward displaying cleavage as her long red polished nails, garnished with diamanté additions reached down to fix the strap on her sling back high heeled sandals. It was early summer.

Introducing myself, I said that I understood she was coming to an appointment with me in a CAMHS (child and adolescent mental health service) because .... but before I could finish, she broke in to tell me that she had been to therapy many times, it was useless and that she had a borderline personality disorder. I asked her if she could say more, to explain to me what she understood that to mean. She glowered at me, told me I must be thick, and why had she come to see a stupid therapist if I didn't know that. She then said she also had bipolar disorder and needed medication for it.

Looking at her scars, I said she was bringing evidence about how much pain she had endured. She fixed me with a glaring look and told me loudly not to stare at her and to mind my own business. It was impossible not to see the injuries unless I covered my eyes or turned my head and looked away. I was stuck. She made it impossible not to see her scars yet told me it was my fault if I saw them. I commented that I had to look but not see. This encounter gave me the experience of feeling like I was being made to 'turn a blind eye' – an accusation that was made against carers and professionals. Attempt by care staff and social workers to notice what the young women were doing and trying to get them to stop provoked an 'it's my choice' response from them. In fact, they were showing them through their actions the pain they endured but demanding at the same time that you do not see it or act on it.

Many of the young people I meet today in clinical settings revel in having been given the label of Borderline Personality Disorder. Like the label victim, they wear it like a badge or pass that gives them leave to behave in particular ways that 'other people don't like' and for which they take no responsibility because they were 'ill' or exploited. With both these labels, they appeared to have no interest in understanding what the label meant or to feel unhappy or discontent with the behaviours they described.

Of particular interest were the types of behaviours these young people were referred for – often self-harming, impulsive, risky, and vulnerable to sexual abuse and exploitation. They are the ones who are likely to be seen to need therapy but unable to engage in formal clinical interventions. These clients often exhibited qualities that appeared to demonstrate a narrative identity rather than an integrated personality. What I mean by that is they tell you about their characteristics rather than beginning to form an actual relationship with you, almost using the narrative as a way to control the relationship. For the worker, it is often so difficult to interject a thought or different idea or ask a curious question. They describe a powerless set of life circumstances in a manner that takes complete control of the space and of the interaction.

This dynamic contradiction is an element of child sexual exploitation and sometimes of the responses of those with responsibility to care for them. These young people feel themselves to be powerless in all manner of ways while at the same time communicating by impact what being controlled feels like. The worker experiences becoming the one who feels powerless.

This Borderline Personality Disorder, a term not often used professionally with young adults, was a diagnosis that Sylvia herself found online and wore proudly as a label. It could more helpfully be understood as what Kernberg (1975) described as a borderline personality organisation. He considered this a broader construct rather than a specific disorder. He suggested that this organisation was a distortion in reality perception rather than the actual loss of contact with reality seen in psychosis. In this way, he reflected that it was an immature and maladaptive defensive organisation offering the person ways of regulating emotion including poor impulse control, low anxiety tolerance, and breakthroughs of 'primary process' thinking, i.e., disordered thinking.

In the same way, Masterson (1972) emphasised how those children who go on to develop a borderline personality disorder have internalised foundational relationship patterns from their interactions with their primary caregivers and formed representations of others who withdraw or attack in response to the child's legitimate expressions of needs and often affects of big or anxious emotions. Adler and Buie (1979) describe this as a deficit in 'evocative object constancy'. They suggest that it is the inability to self-soothe by drawing on memories, images, or experiences with soothing others. They hypothesised that this deficit emerges from childhood experiences with unempathic/unavailable, or abusive parents, who fail to help their children regulate their affects, and ultimately to learn to do so on their own.

These un-empathic, unavailable parents who turned a blind eye to the needs and distress of their babies have been lodged inside these young adults and get re-enacted with adults in the present who are charged with a parental role.

The risk for staff and organisations

The perversity of the system as it exists today is that the organisational imperatives, avoiding risk or blame often mitigate against practices that are in the best interest of the young people and their life trajectories.

In my work consulting to residential units for adolescents, many of the young people are either referred because of, or demonstrate the characteristics of young people involved in child sexual exploitation or child criminal exploitation. They are unable to live in families and previous interventions have not been successful. One problem for staff and residential organisations is the repetition and re-enactments of inappropriate crossing of generational lines prominent in the early developmental experiences of some of these young people. When this has been a sexual abrogation of generational roles, the result is often an over sexualised presentation by the young person. In discussions about sexual exploitation, the young person's behaviour is often described as seductive. In fact, groomers often describe the young women in this way as a means to shift responsibility to the young person rather than themselves.

It is, in many cases, an accurate description, but it remains a description and does not explain such behaviour. These, most often young women, latch onto young attractive male staff members and test boundaries through physical proximity or, more recently, the use of social media to pry or intrude into the personal life of these staff. In the first instance, the staff member might feel flattered or made to feel special or better than the other staff. More personal information is often disclosed as the staff strive to be a friend rather than some crinkly old and out of touch person. This unintended boundary confusion maintains the phantasy for the young person of their specialness and denies generational differences. Un-reflected upon, this can, in fact, lead to inappropriate relationships between staff and residents and the need for rigorous safeguarding procedures to ensure the safety of the young people. Tragically, there are people who take up these jobs to gain access to these vulnerable young people. They need to be identified and dealt with using the full power of the law.

However, it is also too often the case that when the staff member who has been the object of a young person's interest becomes aware of what is happening through supervision, training, etc., and re-establishes a clearer boundary this shift can be experienced quickly and painfully by the young person as a rejection or abandonment, echoing the experience of an earlier parent. The young person easily feels humiliated or pushed away. Having not worked through this earlier confusion or loss of boundary, the young person, now often in grievance mode, makes a complaint against the staff member, who due to safeguarding policies, must be quickly suspended during the intense investigation. Often, when the dust settles, and particularly if the young person has a repeating pattern of allegations, there is a residual anxiety about the quality of care being provided – a mirror of earlier anxiety about the quality of inappropriate relationships that originally brought the young person into care – and there is often a breakdown meeting requested.

Both the social workers involved, and the organisation have 'good reason' to want to move the young person. The social workers to take action or be seen to take action to protect the young person and to avoid being blamed if something further happened. The residential unit because, this might impact on ratings given by the office for standards in education, children's services, and skills (OFSTED) or placing authorities. Both want to move the young person on to avoid other unfounded allegations and are certainly unlikely to fight for them to stay.

On occasion, there are staff who actually cross sexual boundaries and need to be dealt with as predators. But often, it is the repetition of inappropriate maintenance of generational boundaries from their earlier life. Sadly, this can leak into current relationships and lead to repeating breakdown of what was intended as protective care. Grievance can become a container of the negative. While a process of grief leads to mourning and emergence from loss, grievance, especially stemming from early parental loss or care, may lead to the frozen deadened entanglement with the loss.

Another example of how experiences of inappropriate early parental boundaries can get mirrored in the system is the use of Deprivation of Liberty Orders. (DOL Gov.UK 2023). A deprivation of liberty order makes it lawful for a child to be deprived of their liberty. The court authorises the order, and any restrictions are set out clearly in the order. Children of any age, subject to this order, generally require high levels of care and supervision. This means that a child subject to a deprivation of liberty order will likely also be on a Care Order and be placed in a children's home. These orders are often instigated when the young person remains at risk but is being discharged from inpatient hospital care. In 2021, there was a dramatic increase in the use of these orders – a 462% increase since 2018. This likely equates, with the closure of 16 secure children's homes since 2002 (Gov.UK/Ofsted 2021). It seems that with the use of this order there is a desire that an ordinary residential unit can be made secure without the necessary physical boundaries, such as security doors that prevent the young person from leaving.

Yet while increased high staff ratios and mandated restraint training stand alongside deprivation of liberty planning, even this cannot ensure the young people remain on site and safe. The problem remains that many young people involved in sexual and criminal exploitation see the workers as the bad guys and work hard to run away from the homes and to the groomers and gang leaders. Despite the discourse of young people needing to be near their families and communities, without resource intensive therapeutic work with the family it is often only the geographical distance that offers some psychic separation. Ironically, these orders re-create the lack of safe boundaries that were part of early parenting. The staff can then be seen as neglectful and powerless parents who are ineffectual at keeping their children safe or turn a blind eye while abuse is happening. Attempts to safeguard persistently risky residents through restraint, even when restraining techniques are ethically and scrupulously applied,[1] can come to be experienced by some staff and young people like an echo of the physical control of early abusive authoritarian parents. The result can too often be blame and breakdown. Having to start again in new placements can leave these young people less safe. Working to hold on to these extremely difficult young people could be one of the most helpful ways of challenging sexual exploitation.

Adolescents generally, and this population of young people especially, are rarely easy to engage in therapy since they experience the therapist as dangerous or useless and never make it to a consulting room. Instead, training the staff of residential homes to recognise these complex unconscious processes and the powerful and sometimes toxic feelings and behaviours that get evoked when living with some of these traumatised young people may offer a more effective route to change. Valuing the work of front-line staff and investing in intensive packages of care that actually address the challenges of building reparative relationships must be prioritised. It is only when trust begins to be established and the young person starts to experience a different kind of adult care that is not exploitative or abusive that any meaningful change in their personality structure can begin. But as young people are in flight or fight mode, this is more challenging than policymakers suggest. Just 'being nice but being firm' is not as easy as it sounds. It goes unrecognised by many organisations and funding bodies how slow this process of change can be. The model of telling young people they are victims and 'empowering' them can only go so far. It is not easy to intervene. Often, these young people are excellent at re-producing psychobabble or internet speak. But reiterating other people's insights is not the same as integrating them into the self.

None of the illustrations used are of actual people or incidents. Rather, they are an amalgam of aspects of many exploited young people and care situations that I have come into contact with over the years. I never cease to be amazed at the dedication and endless patience of the workers and the tenacity of the young people whose situations need more understanding.

Note

1 Minimising and Managing Physical Restraint (MMPR): Safeguarding Processes, Governance Arrangements, and Roles and Responsibilities Ministry of Justice, National Offender Management Service, and Youth Justice Board for England and Wales. Published 9 July 2012, https://assets.publishing.service.gov.uk/media/5a802021ed915d74e33f8980/minimising-managing-physical-restraint.pdf

References

Adler, G. and Buie, D. (1979) *Aloneness and borderline psychopathology: The possible relevance of child development issues.* The International Journal of Psychoanalysis, 60(1) 83–96.

Basch, M. (1983) *Empathic understanding: A review of the concept and some theoretical considerations.* Journal of the American Psychoanalytic Association, 31(1) 101–126.

Bower, M. and Solomon, R. (2018) *Cruel Protectors: Understanding Sexual Exploitation* Chap 11. In Bower, M. and Solomon, R. (Eds) *What Social Workers Need to Know: A Psychoanalytic Approach.* London, Routledge.

Britton, R. (1994) *The blindness of the seeing eye: inverse symmetry as a defence against reality.* Psychoanalytic Inquiry, 14(3) 365–378.

Canham, H. (2002) *Group and gang states of mind.* Journal of Child Psychotherapy, 28:2, 113–127, DOI: 10.1080/00754170210143753

Cregeen, S. (2008) *Workers, groups and gangs: Consultation to residential adolescent teams.* Journal of Child Psychotherapy, 34 172–189.

DfE Gov.UK July 2014 (last updated 2018) *Promoting the education of looked-after and previously looked-after children* https://assets.publishing.service.gov.uk/

media/5a9015d4e5274a5e67567fbe/Promoting_the_education_of_looked-after_children_and_previously_looked-after_children.pdf

Freud, S (1914) 'Remembering, Repeating and Working-Through' (Standard Edition, XII, pp. 147–56)

Glasser, M (1979) *Aspects of the Role of Aggression in the Perversions*. In I. Rosen (Ed) (1998) Sexual Deviations. Oxford: OUP.

Gov.UK/Ofsted (2021) *National Statistics, Main findings: children's social care in England* https://www.gov.uk/government/statistics/childrens-social-care-data-in-england-2022/main-findings-childrens-social-care-in-england-2022

Gov.UK/Ofsted (2023) *Placing Children: deprivation of liberty orders (guidance)* https://www.gov.uk/government/publications/placing-children-deprivation-of-liberty-orders/placing-children-deprivation-of-liberty-orders#:~:text=A%20DoL%20order%20makes%20it,levels%20of%20care%20and%20supervision.

Jankowitz, S.E. (2018) *The Victim-Perpetrator Paradigm. The Order of Victimhood. Palgrave Studies in Compromise after Conflict*. London, Palgrave Macmillan, Cham.

Joseph, B. (1982) *Addiction to near-death*. Int Journal of Psychoanalysis, 63 449–56. PMID: 7152808.

Kernberg, O. (1975) *Borderline Conditions and Pathological Narcissism*. Maryland USA, J. Aronson Press.

Masterson, J. (1972) *Treatment of the Borderline Adolescent: A Developmental Approach*. New York USA, Brunner/Mazel. (Reprinted 1986 Brunner-Routledge.)

Stubley, J. in *Ask Annalisa Barbieri www.theguardian.com* 12 May 2023.

6

LOST AND FOUND AND THE NEED FOR BELONGING

Exploring the risk of exploitation for young people living on the edge of care

Alison Roy

Introduction and context

When I was asked to write this chapter, my first thoughts were that I wouldn't know where to begin. However, as I started to recall my encounters with looked after and adopted children and young people over the 20+ years of working in children's mental health services, and in community settings, I realised how many of them had indeed experienced exploitation in some form or other and how lost and disorientated they were and felt. It is this experience of being and feeling lost that I would like to write about when thinking about exploitation and how in trying to understand and represent a "lost" young person's feelings and experiences, I too found that I became isolated and exposed and even felt rather lost as I struggled to find my voice within the professional network.

These young people on the edge of care or being cared for can exist on the fringes of society, and it can take a crisis before anyone really takes notice of them. They are vulnerable to exploitation because they can so easily be overlooked and because they continually struggle to locate or place themselves or understand their own history/story. Their rootlessness, being blown here, there, and everywhere, is perhaps a result of being uprooted too many times and becoming familiar with the experience of rejection and of not being "chosen".

I am also writing this within the context of living in a changed world. I refer not only to the 2020 Covid pandemic but also to the way that technology has altered society and social norms and presented additional or new risks and challenges for us all, but especially our young people. Smartphones, for example, have significantly influenced the way most humans communicate and connect (or disconnect) with each other – through the touch of a button or the swipe of

DOI: 10.4324/9781003020370-6

a screen. These devices have redefined our public but also private and intimate spaces and the way we communicate and can also intrude into our places of safety. Many of the connections young people make with others now happen online through social networks, forums, and other virtual meeting places where it can be hard to monitor what is really going on.

Unfortunately, it isn't only the way young people meet and communicate that has changed, but the way that they present themselves to the world. This way of being seen and known on a public forum may expose them to further risks and much can be learned about a child or young person through their online presence and profile.

For children and young people who are "looked after" – in foster care, residential homes, or are living within adoptive families, there are additional risks. Contact with birth parents before the arrival of social media would usually have been managed carefully and supervised. For adopted children, this contact may well have been in the form of a letter through a letter box. Since there appear to be few agreed rules, boundaries, or safety checks in place for social media platforms, understandably curious children and young people who want to know more about their birth family can use these platforms to find information without those who care for them being aware of it.

This form of unsupervised contact poses a number of risks and dilemmas for parents and professionals but also even sometimes for the birth parents themselves. Young people in the care system have usually experienced significant losses and potentially a number of placement disruptions. These disruptions or ruptures will have affected their capacity to build healthy attachments as written about by Hindle and Shulman (2008), Emmanuel (2002), and Lanyado (2004, 2017).

In addition to these more obvious adversities, it is the sad fact that many of these young people have learned to view themselves as transferable or marketable "goods". I have worked with adopted young people in groups where this is a key theme. They describe themselves as children and how they would have done almost anything to be wanted or "chosen". One young woman told me that as a child, she tried her hardest to look "cute" when her photo was taken for an adoption recruitment event. She also remembers feeling confused, unlovable, and unwanted while doing her best to smile.

Many of these children have, therefore, unfortunately, learned very early on in their lives, how to sell themselves and can follow others indiscriminately in order not to be left behind or risk being/feeling unwanted. Those of us who have worked in children's services or children's centres have all come across children who will take a stranger's hand, sit on their knee, or ask to be taken home. This is then a "double deprivation" as described by Henry (1974) or even "triple deprivation" Emanuel (2002).

These formative childhood experiences and resulting behaviours introduce a level of vulnerability into these young people's lives which can unfortunately increase the risk to them of exploitation and make it much more complicated for them to understand the difference between good and harmful relationships.

There are a number of young adults who have shared their stories on social media who describe how loneliness and feeling different to their peers was a contributing factor to their risk-taking behaviours. This was certainly the case for the young people who came through our specialist adoption service I co-founded called AdCAMHS (Roy et. al, 2017, Roy 2020).

Jackie Kay, the Scottish poet laureate and an adopted adult, has written about her life and experience as an adoptee in *Red Dust Road* (2010). The book describes her journey to finding her birth parents, but it also describes how, as a child and young person, she felt lonely and different despite being loved by her adoptive parents.

"My mum all those years ago sensed a child who had been adopted was also a child who could feel terribly hurt .... no matter how much she loved me ... there is still a windy place right at the core of my heart. The windy place is like Wuthering Heights, out on the open moors, rugged and wild and free and lonely ...."

Another young woman I worked with articulated her reasons for remaining in an abusive but also exploitative relationship because, she said, it was a relief for her to be "wanted" but also not to have her own troubling thoughts – in other words, to not have to endure having her own "windy and lonely place". Someone else made all the decisions for her and took over the control of her life. She did not want to be left with her own thoughts or to have "a mind of One's own", Waddell (1998). She described herself as numb and "sleepwalking" into a "dark place", but every time she woke up, she had to work hard to find a way to go back to sleep again.

Understanding why

Being awake and alive, seeing who she had become and what she had suffered, felt unbearable. However, when a genuine offer of "care" and a more consistent relationship presented itself, it felt too exposing and dangerous for her. The possibility of intimacy, however attractive, threatened her defences – her very survival and challenged her so-called pain relief and addictive behaviours. The result was that she continued to return to the abusive relationship and moved on to other gang members who continued to exploit and abuse her.

Many young people in similar situations to this young woman and her patterns of relating have lost their sense of themselves as social and moral beings who feel. They have taught themselves how to become numb and to ignore not only their feelings but also their desires and their wish to be valued and cared for.

Rather than feeling secure in their attachments, they feel activated by them, confused, distressed, and often afraid. This leads to a disconnect from those "people who do relationships" as one young person described it, and they try to find others who they perceive as being more like themselves. Unfortunately, these "others" are also more likely to engage in destructive and spoiling behaviours (Meltzer, 1986).

Chris Scanlon and John Adlam's latest book – "Psycho-social Explorations of Trauma, Exclusion and Violence ...." Scanlon and Adlam (2022) explores the psycho-social traumatisation of being excluded or "un-housed" and how the experience of being on the outside and the resulting feeling of shame, creates a risk or further exclusion. They argue that a lack of inclusion and protection from our political and social system potentially sets these young people up to be exploited.

They quote Gilligan:

> I have yet to see a serious act of violence that was not provoked by the experience of feeling shamed and humiliated, disrespected, and ridiculed, and that did not represent the attempt to prevent or undo this "loss of face ...."
>
> *(Gilligan 1996, p 110)*

Without a place – their own space, where they can be thought about and protected, these "outside" young people can easily be picked up by unscrupulous individuals and recruited into gangs. They will also potentially learn how to recruit and exploit others further down the line (Cregeen 2017).

In the writing of my book about adoption (*A For Adoption*, Roy 2020), I interviewed a number of young people, some of whom had themselves been exploited, in order to understand more about why they run away. I concluded that:

> Sometimes the running is simply a way of communicating distress. Running away presents new and increased risks, which parents and professionals find difficult to deal with. Even those who seem relatively "settled" in their adolescence speak about times when they need to run away .... running can take young people into alien and unsafe environments where they risk losing more than the freedom to make their own decisions. Adopted young people have had at least one experience of being thrust into an alien environment, so it may be that running away holds a certain attraction and familiarity for them or that something is being reenacted through the act of running.
>
> *(Roy 2020, p. 72)*

Those who have managed to make some sense of their dysfunctional patterns in relationships have described to me how their instinctive drive to run and hide, coupled with their desire to find their birth family or others like them, predictably led them not to safety but into danger. I describe this drive or desire as "the call of the wild". It is important that parents, carers, and professionals understand the significance of this call if they are to help their young people understand how they are being pulled in different directions and the risks as they seek to work out who they are and where they belong.

The differences between groups and gangs are written about by Bion (1962b) and others (Foulkes 1983, 1990; Hopper 1997). They make a distinction between the group and "groupishness" (1990) versus the gang or gang like behaviour. These insights can help us understand how vulnerable young people who struggle with their own internal gang are more easily targeted.

Bion (1967) used his experiences in the First World War to understand the different behaviours humans will use in order to protect themselves and survive including blindly following orders without thinking for themselves. Drawing upon the work of Bion, Rosenfeld (1971) and Melzer (1968) further develop the hypothesis that there exists in the life of the mind and the group (or gang) an "internal establishment" – a highly organised agency with a protected and restricted way of living or being.

As these young people I am describing have either lost their early attachment figures (Bowlby, 1973, 1980, 1988) or never felt securely attached in the first place, they will have very little sense of what home and safety feels like. Their experience and associated feelings of being abandoned by their primary caregivers – the rejected, hurt, and angry feelings can begin to take on a life or shape of their own. Meltzer (1968) highlights the destructiveness of these feelings and the internal forces, "gang" or "establishment" and the pursuit for control through the use of lies and violence. Curiosity, questioning, and truthfulness – or having a mind, is not permitted.

This behaviour becomes more readily accepted by gang members and can be very difficult to challenge or shift. Bion used the terms "beta-elements" (1962/1965) and "inchoate elements" (1967) to describe those feelings which become fragmented – the elements that cannot be processed. These are not linked to the development of thinking apparatus, or of having a mind that can tolerate frustration. They can only be dealt with by expulsion which leads to acting out – to "not-thinking". He also referred to destructive attacks made by the patient on anything or anyone with the function of linking and thinking (1959).

"In contrast with the alpha-elements the beta-elements are not felt to be phenomena, but things in themselves" (p. 6).

I am reminded her of the well-known children's book by Maurice Sendak, *Where the Wild Things Are* (1963), where Max is taken over by wild feelings or "things". His mother calls him "Wild Thing" and sends him to bed without his supper.

Thankfully for Max, his mother (although she doesn't feature much in the book in person) does find a way to make sense of her own and her son's wild feelings, having been sorely tested, and provides him with his supper – the good feed or breast (Klein 1959a, 1959b). Max's appetite and yearning are satiated, he knows that he is thought about, will be provided for despite his wild feelings and finds his way "home" or back to himself.

This level of containment and understanding facilitates a transformation of the monstrous or "wild things" (the gang) within him. Whereas young people who find themselves in the grip of a gang which may mirror their own internal "establishment" feel controlled from both within and without. It can feel to them that there is no escape from their monstrous feelings and so they become concretely stuck in a very wild, inhospitable, and dangerous place, fuelled by their belief that they are fundamentally bad. The "wild thing" within will require significant containment and transformation (Bion, 1961) before healthier ways of relating can become possible.

Getting young people to place of safety where they can begin to do this transformative work and think for themselves is a huge challenge for those willing to try. It isn't surprising that many of those on the edge of care struggle to risk meaningful connections, are driven by feelings of shame and guilt and start to become less visible to the professional network around them and are then even harder to reach. It is worth noting that professionals and carers need to be supported to acknowledge and understand this disconnect they may feel from the young person but also towards each other, making it difficult to work constructively as a group.

Connections lost and found

Ironically, it is the connecting "lines" of phones and trains that are used to exploit disconnected and fragmented young people. The term "County Lines" refers to the way that phone and train lines are used to transport mostly drugs and money between different counties. The young people involved in this process are usually given little information about who they are meeting and where they will end up, but they continue to be exploited and exposed in this way in order to extend the reach and potency of the gang. If these young people are caught, they pay the price for possession of drugs, money, or weapons, but the ring leaders will do their utmost to remain anonymous and "disconnected". The phones that are used are usually old Nokia phones that can't be traced or tracked unlike smartphones. Direct train routes provide easy connections between counties meaning that young people cross over into counties or territories where they won't be known and are less easily "found" or intercepted.

A number of lines are being crossed here, physically, and geographically but also legally, meaning that young people are made to feel afraid of speaking out, asking for help, or questioning those exploiting them. A boundary is also being crossed personally, morally, and psychologically in that any self-protectiveness or showing care and respect for others or the self is discouraged or completely dispensed with. The focus instead becomes survival and on not getting caught.

I wish to refer here to an adopted young man of 15. I will call him Pete. He was very much on the edge of care in that he no longer lived with his parents, and his numerous foster placements and supported lodgings had broken down. It was feared that he had been targeted by a gang and exploited in exchange for a new phone and a supply of drugs, but he had a number of concerned adults trying to keep their connection with him going. I, too, repeatedly tried to connect with him when he was first referred to me, but he found it incredibly difficult to attend the clinic appointments and appeared to be very much under the control of a gang. He was regularly discussed in numerous professional network meetings, forums, and safeguarding teams or hubs, but no one had really succeeded in getting hold of him.

What I became aware of through my work with Pete was how much time was spent finding him before therapy could even begin. The connective routes established by the gang served to keep him and others like him on the move and out of reach. He (they) always seemed to be one step ahead of us. For Pete, it was a method of avoiding emotional pain, but he was also concretely running from those he owed money to and regularly informed me about the people "after him" – a list which increased with each passing week as did his paranoia and his fear of being caught. It became more difficult for those who were trying to help him to make contact with him and get him to a safer place. Whenever he did make it to see me, he looked agitated, unable to sit still or give me eye contact. However, the connection between Pete's social worker and myself was invaluable in keeping hold of him and giving him an experience of being held in mind Winnicott (1953, 1960) by a thinking couple.

I noted on one session that Pete had a glazed look about him and couldn't focus. I tried to explore with him whether this was to do with using substances or whether he had reached "system overload" as I called it, which led to Pete shutting down emotionally. He did admit to using "weed" to calm him down before his session but could also quickly become volatile when challenged. Safety for both of us became a focus in my conversations with his social worker, in my own supervision and in the network meetings.

I remember on one occasion when Pete was still in a supportive lodgings type placement, his carer brought him to his session and he was openly furious with her, shouting at her and kicking off in the clinic waiting room. It transpired that she had agreed to take him shopping after his therapy, but he had only heard the "shopping" part of the communication and was feeling aggrieved about being coming to the clinic first. He hurled expletives and insults at her but then became distressed when she walked out and drove away, leaving him with me. I risked suggesting that there might be a very small part of him that did want help and had allowed himself to come to therapy and that perhaps he was more cross with himself than his carer. He replied that the part of him who wanted to come was "so small it was microscopic!" He proceeded to name call me his therapist since his carer had moved out of the firing line.

He finally came into the therapy room but paced around the room feeling unable to settle, shouting but holding his head as if in pain every time I spoke. We both survived the experience, mostly through my listening and staying quiet and calm, my reflections or interpretations would not have been received by Pete in such an agitated state. The need to adapt and gauge the temperature in the room was an important and my way of showing Pete that I was listening to him, that I wasn't going to threaten him but nor was I intimidated by him.

The following session, he agreed to come to the clinic with his social worker, who became the main and most successful "taxi service" in getting Pete to his therapy sessions. Once in the room, he became very lucid and started to draw lines over the chalkboard. I asked him to describe what he was drawing and where all these lines were leading to. He seemed confused by what he had drawn, so I suggested that it looked like an impossible maze. He nodded, so I wondered where he would place himself in the mass of lines, speech bubbles, and crossed connections (lines that could easily be rubbed out). He explained that although he was in the picture he couldn't be found. (A bit like the "Where's Wally" books, only his intention was not to be spotted.) A thought I verbalised and asked Pete if he was willing to let me try. He shook his head but added that he had spent most of his life on the run, hiding "bits" of himself in different places. He hadn't known if they would be safe. He concluded by telling me, "There's more, but I can't tell you …"

As I tried to gather up what I could from the fragments or "bits" of Pete's history, I realised that the lost feelings or parts of himself along with his story had over time, become "things in themselves", and had taken on a life of their own. They had "grown teeth and claws", I explained to the professional network.

I felt strongly that Pete had wanted to tell me more about his story but also his current predicament, his fear about himself as bad and the chaos of running from gang to gang. However, after each session, he struggled to come back, and every attended session was followed by one or two missed sessions. It was as if he knew coming to see me would mean facing a painful truth. Significant input from the network was required to "gather him up" and get him to his therapy sessions, his further education course (he had been permanently excluded from school) or his Youth Attending Team (YOT) meetings. On one occasion, Pete informed me that he was on a train and planning to come to his therapy session, but he was running late. I felt that something was wrong and knew he wouldn't make it but hoped that he would. I found myself checking in with reception repeatedly and looking out of the window, feeling a mixture of hopefulness that he might arrive at any moment, which sometimes he did, or a fear that he would be lost forever. It was impossible to get on with other work while waiting for him to arrive. His social worker also reported similar feelings of concern and frustration as he tried to locate Pete, driving to all the usual places where he could be and then persuading him to come.

After his fourth foster placement broke down, Pete was housed in a hostel and was sometimes found to be asleep when the social worker came to collect him. He would arrive in a dishevelled state, late but present. More often than not, however, he was determined to outsmart his social worker and claimed that he didn't need picking up and would make his own way to therapy. I think he genuinely did intend to see me, believing he could decide for himself, but all too often, his sessions were spent on and off the phone updating me on his difficult journey. He had been thrown off the train for not having a ticket or he was on the wrong train – or he didn't know where he was going, or he had to go and see someone first. Sometimes I would hear voices in the background, and there were repeated dramas on route, numerous fallouts with people, usually over the phone, including girlfriends or carers trying to keep tabs on him. Tracking behaviour has become a big part of the exploitation journey, drug running, and gang culture and these vulnerable but also tricky young people allow themselves to be moved around. They are invested in not being found, but the fact that they had a difficult journey right at the start of their lives is in the mix to be thought about. Unfortunately, as I have already discussed, this may also mean that the exploited young person may never really "arrive" – being lost is familiar to them, and they have no way of locating themselves on a map.

I noted that Pete always had more than one phone which I challenged him about. I discussed (and documented) my concerns about exploitation with him, his social worker, and the professional network. Network meetings were often quite emotionally intense occasions where Pete (if he attended) tried to talk his way out of the messes and scrapes he had got himself into or crimes he had committed. Some of the incidents had involved violence or exploitation of others. He would try to deflect or deny the distress he had caused to others and always had a reason why he couldn't do what he was supposed to do. The adults supporting him expressed sadness and disappointment with his attitude and behaviour when they felt they had gone out of their way to help him. What was curious was that despite everything, he was liked, and people wanted to help him. I commented on one occasion that I experienced him as being like a "front of house salesman", he could be charming and was bright and capable, but he was also selling me a version of himself I didn't really believe, and it was very difficult to know what was really going on behind the scenes. He laughed at this analogy but seemed to be observing me closely throughout the rest of the meeting, trying to work me out. He also told numerous lies or stories about himself to others, some about his birth parents which bore very little resemblance to the truth. Little was known about his birth, but his birth mother was known to social care; her life was plagued by abuse, addiction, and violent relationships and she had been a child in care herself.

Understanding or at least recognising patterns in behaviour and naming our feelings where possible is an important part of the work with young people on the very edge of care and on the fringes of society. The usual boundaries such as clear session times and not being under the influence of substances can be difficult to enforce.

I found that if I did try to enforce "rules" or boundaries, I could lose the precious and precarious connection with Pete. I also felt responsible for the loss of connection and for keeping him safe despite the huge challenges involved in doing this. It was important to acknowledge if he did arrive (on the wrong day, for example) that he had battled with his internal and external gang to make it to the clinic. I would usually try to see him if only briefly. Opinion was divided about this in network meetings and in my discussions in supervision, which meant that I also felt that I was testing boundaries and, at times, that I was being unfairly judged and scrutinised.

Getting the network together proved to be complicated in the early days and finding a shared time when everyone could meet was a major challenge. It was as if we were all living in different time zones and could not synchronise our clocks. These practical difficulties could be understood as manifestations of the emotional experience of fragmentation and of how it feels to be with Pete. As a group, we began to recognise the importance of owning and speaking about these feelings of helplessness and a fear of getting things wrong or losing touch with Pete.

Creativity and transformation

Over decades of working with some of the most hard-to-reach, traumatised and disconnected individuals, I have come to understand that the ability to adapt is key. This doesn't mean that safety and boundaries are dispensed with, but it is the adaptability and the willingness to think (and interpret) on the move, which can begin to make a difference for these young people. They have very little sense of what it means to trust, and the system they operate within lacks a cohesive social structure or moral code. They are, therefore, suspicious of rules and boundaries, and it can take a while for them to acknowledge the safety they provide.

In addition to adaptability is the importance of being part of a professional community. It's not possible to keep these young people safe on your own. Working closely and supportively with the network can and does make a difference as this helps the young person to remain visible. In Pete's case, I continued to support the professional network after the therapy had ended, encouraging them as a group to stay focused on finding a different and more creative approach to managing the risks. This included understanding Pete's history and the context of the "stories" he told and understanding more about his relationships and what they meant to him rather than seeking to scrutinise and control all his comings and goings which only exacerbated his feelings of paranoia.

Before becoming a child psychotherapist, I directed a community arts project for young people Not in Education or Employment (NEET). On one occasion, a member of the group turned up for a group art session carrying a handgun which he casually placed on the desk. I was rather thrown by this and immediately phoned the community policeman who was linked to the project to get his advice on how to manage this situation. He was alarmed but also reluctant to call armed policemen who would be likely to arrive at the arts project imminently. The project was a safe haven for excluded young people on the fringes of society and we both feared in terms of risk that the presence of armed police would affect the stability and safety of the wider group.

He asked me questions I couldn't answer about whether the gun was real, loaded, etc., so I agreed that I would try to have a conversation with the young person before notifying the police in a more official capacity. I also agreed to complete a risk assessment of the situation and call him back.

The young person who was 17 at the time, had had periods of being homeless and accommodated in and out of young offender's institutions. He was regularly on the run, but I had discovered that he was also a talented artist and a good photographer. He had produced art pieces with me and the group for arts events and communicated something of his story through his art. I asked him to give me the gun which he did without hesitation. I then attempted to talk to him about the meaning of the gun, its purpose, and my confusion about why it had been brought into our safe space. I wondered what needed to happen in order to keep him and others in the group safe. He insisted that the gun wasn't loaded but that he carried it around for protection because someone was "after him". His fears which on first impressions appeared to be rather paranoid, had grown from a very real place of being continually hurt and let down by those he should have been able to trust. His sense was that no-one was looking out for him. He agreed to leave his gun with me in exchange for a camera which offered him a different kind of security. The gun was disposed of, and he was allowed to take the camera home with him and around the town to photograph graffiti or anything that caught his eye. I suggested that it might also help him to describe more of his own story. This was a transformative experience for him and although weeks later, he sold the camera, we were able to use the images he took and do some thinking as a group about how it can be possible to transform violence and hurt into ideas about survival and resilience. The phrase "a camera for your gun" took on its own creative meaning within the group.

Many of the adopted young people who came through our specialist adoption mental health service in East Sussex (AdCAMHS) benefitted from the opportunity to be creative and to share their stories in more unconventional settings. One of these was a young person (Nya) who was 14 when she first came to see me. She was known to the police as one of the "ring leaders" of a local gang who they believed was dealing drugs and engaging in exploitation and theft, but they didn't have much evidence to go on. They hoped that Nya, as a minor, would be able to give them useful information, but this had not been forthcoming. Members of the professional network supporting her, and her family were all exasperated with her as well as concerned about her. They couldn't understand why she had felt so drawn to the gang. At school, she had been caught dealing drugs to friends and was excluded. She had also been accused of exploiting vulnerable people in the community and had been arrested on a number of occasions for petty crime and low-level aggression. She would also disappear for days on end.

Nya's early childhood was traumatic, and she experienced physical and sexual abuse. When I first met her, she seemed unavailable emotionally (possibly under the influence of cannabis and/or alcohol) and in constant conflict with her adoptive mother who described how Nya had been reasonably well behaved, although feisty until she reached puberty. It was at this point that she was allegedly assaulted by a so-called male friend. When she tried to tell the school staff about it, they hadn't believed her, possibly because she was someone who they described as "creating a drama" and had also been challenging in class. This is a familiar pattern and worth being aware of. Predatory adults and peers can work out those who are unlikely to be believed and are, therefore, more easily exploited. Her behaviour significantly deteriorated after the assault and she started to miss school and "hang out" with people who were threatening to others, but as she explained, "they will stand by me if anyone tries to hurt me". This is crucial. I have encountered a number of young people who, when they feel that professionals and/or parental figures fail to protect them from harm, will find their own version of a protective group or gang.

Nya always arrived at her session furious. This was either with the police who on occasion appeared to have been heavy handed with her, with her peer group or with her adoptive parents. I had the sense that being in close proximity to others was frightening for her, but she masked her fear by projecting it into others or by provoking them into aggression towards her.

She told me very clearly in our first session (with her adoptive mother present) that she couldn't be in a room with me on her own and if this happened, she would just run. Initially, we tried meeting for five minutes on our own but with her mother coming in at the start. After the first month, we moved to ten minutes, and eventually, she stayed for fifteen minutes each week.

We also agreed some boundaries around her drug use and turning up to sessions. I then negotiated a longer session and was helped by the family dog. We would begin the session in the clinic room but then move outdoors walking the dog (even in the middle of winter). I talked mostly to the dog about my concerns for Nya and wondered out loud how we would keep her safe and help her to trust me. I reflected on the unfairness of what had happened to her and her feeling that she hadn't been believed and taken seriously.

I remember on one session sitting on a park bench after a recent court case when Nya had been charged with theft which (in her mind) had been taken very seriously by the police, whereas the assault she had suffered had not been properly investigated and had instead been disregarded. The family dog who was normally lively, sat still and close to her with his head resting on her lap. She stroked him gently which I hadn't seen her do before. These little shifts where tenderness became possible, felt deeply significant and represented the beginning of a shift in Nya's internal world and the gang's hold over her. Although she could only allow herself to give and receive small amounts of kindness and empathy, she continued to see me and risked a deeper connection with me, her attendance improving with each month that went by.

Despite being vulnerable, Nya was tall and striking, and appeared streetwise, feisty, and strong. She had broken down doors, punched holes in walls, and fought off policemen, but she also had a soft side and an affinity for animals. She once talked me through the process of wrestling with and then "breaking in" a wild horse. During our work, I sensed that she was wrestling with the hurting and wild part of herself, but she also found the strength to fight the external gang and started waking up from her sleep.

Conclusion

When a young person really decides to fight for themselves and their future – things will inevitably change. The hold of the internal gang diminishes as does the grip of the external gang. However, they may also become more threatening to the young person. In Nya's case, members of the gang continued to threaten her and her family, but as the hold of the internal "gang" Meltzer (1968) weakened, so did the power of the external gang. We weathered these storms together with the help of the professional network. I also supported parents to think about their capacity to protect Nya and themselves. Nya's ability to tolerate boundaries increased and she started to acknowledge that she wanted to be with me in a safe and secure space and her psychotherapy sessions moved to the therapy room.

By the time our therapy ended, Nya was free of the gang and her scars, physical (such as cuts and burns) as well as emotional were beginning to heal. She even offered to come back to speak to parent groups I was running, about gangs and running away how to notice the signs. She was clear that she wanted others to learn from her experience of running away and feeling stuck in a cycle of exploitation and abuse.

For Pete, although he cut his therapy short, he attended 15 sessions in all, one for every year of his life and started to make a few good friends (including a girlfriend) outside the gang and despite continued dramas and settled into a new supported living placement. In my experience then, I have witnessed how psycBergehoanalytic psychotherapy can be a powerful tool for treating these young people. The therapeutic relationship or alliance invites them to connect with someone who is consistently available to them and for them, providing live company, Alvarez (1992). Even young people who appear "lost" can be "found" through the experience of being with someone who understands them and the powerful or "wild" forces at work within them, often pulling them in different directions and getting them into all kinds of trouble. It is an approach which requires creativity and adaptability, and it takes time. It may involve a re-setting of more realistic boundaries, but it can support better risk management and care planning as it keeps the young person and their history or story right at the centre of the work, placing them firmly back on the map.

Sendak's Max, after the excitement of his dream, wanted to be where someone loved him best of all (Sendak 1963).

References

Alvarez, A. (1992). *Live Company*. London and New York, Tavistock/Routledge.

Bion, W. (1959). *Attacks on Linking. International Journal of Psychoanalysis*, 40 (5–6) p 308

Bion, W. (1961). *Experiences in Groups and Other Papers*. London, Tavistock.

Bion, W. (1967). *A theory of thinking*. International Journal of Psychoanalysis, 43(4–5); reprinted in *Second Thoughts* (1967).

Bion, W. (1962). *Learning from Experience*.; Reprinted London, Heinemann Medical Books, Karnac, 1984.

Bion, W. (1967). *Second Thoughts: Selected Papers on Psychoanalysis* (1984). London, Karnac (Books) Ltd. (Originally composed between 1950 and 1962).

Bowlby, J. (1973). *Attachment and Loss. Vol. 2 Separation: Anxiety and Anger*. New York, NY Basic Books.

Bowlby, J. (1980). *Attachment and Loss*. London, Hogarth Press: Institute of Psychoanalysis.

Bowlby, J. (1988). *A Secure Base: Parent-Child Attachment and Healthy Human Development*. New York, Basic Books.

Cregeen, S. (2017). *A place within the heart: Finding a home with parental objects*. Journal of Child Psychotherapy, 43(2), 159–174.

Emanuel, L. (2002, August). *Deprivation x three: The contribution of organizational dynamics to the "triple deprivation" of looked after children*. Journal of Child Psychotherapy, 28(2), 163–179.

Foulkes, S.H. (1983). *Introduction to Group-Analytic Psychotherapy: Studies in the Social Integration of Individuals and Groups*. London, Maresfield Reprints.

Foulkes, S.H. (1990). *Selected Papers: Psychoanalysis and Group Analysis*. London, Karnac.

Gilligan, J. (1996). *Violence, Our Deadly Epidemic and Its Causes*. New York and London, Putnam.

Henry, G. (1974). *Doubly deprived*. Journal of Child Psychotherapy, 3(4), 15–28.

Hindle, D. & Shulman, G. (2008). *The Emotional Experience of Adoption – a Psychoanalytic Perspective*. Abingdon, Routledge.

Hopper, E. (1997). *Traumatic experience in the unconscious life of groups: A fourth basic assumption*. London, Group Analysis, December 1, 30(4), 439–470. https://doi.org/10.1177/0533316497304002

Kay, J. (2010) *Red Dust Road*: London, Picador. Second edition (2017) Picador Classic, paperback.

Klein, M. (1959a). *Our Adult World and Its Roots in Infancy in (1975) The Writings of Melanie Klein Vol 3*. London, Routledge.

Klein, M. (1959b). *The Psychoanalysis of Children*. London, Hogarth Press.

Lanyado, M. (2004). *The Presence of the Therapist: Treating Childhood Trauma*. London, Routledge.

Lanyado, M. (2017). *Transforming Despair to Hope. Reflections on the Psychotherapeutic Process with Severely Neglected and Traumatised Children*. London, Routledge.

Meltzer, D. (1968). *Terror, persecution, dread: A dissection of paranoid anxieties*. The International Journal of Psychoanalysis, 49(2–3), 396–401.

Rosenfeld, H. (1971). *A clinical approach to the psychoanalytic theory of the life and death instincts: An investigation into the aggressive aspects of narcissism*. The International Journal of Psychoanalysis, 52(2), 169–178.

Roy, A. (2020). *A For Adoption*. Oxon, Routledge.

Roy, A., Thomas, C. & Simmonds, J. (2017). *Adoption Support: Integrating Social Work and Therapeutic Services – the AdCAMHS Model*. London, Coram BAAF Briefing series.

Scanlon, C. & Adlam, J. (2022). *Psycho-Social Explorations of Trauma, Exclusion and Violence: Un-Housed Minds and Inhospitable Environments*. London, Routledge.

Sendak, M. (1963). *Where the Wild Things Are*. New York, NY, Harper & Row.

Waddell, M. (1998). *Inside Lives: Psychoanalysis and the Growth of the Personality*. London, Duckworth & Co. Ltd.

Winnicott, D.W. (1953). *Transitional objects and transitional phenomena – a study of the first not-me*. International Journal of Psychoanalysis, 34, 89–97.

Winnicott, D.W. (1960). *The theory of the parent-infant relationship*. International Journal of Psychoanalysis, 41, 585–595.

7

A FATHER IN MIND

The importance of considering 'paternal functions' when caring for vulnerable young women who are at risk of sexual exploitation

Robin Solomon

After participating in many case discussions and reading many files about complex adolescents who were seen to be vulnerable to exploitation, I became interested in the lack of visibility of the role that fathers played in the early experience of these mostly young women. The dominant narrative is often focused on disturbance or neglect in the mother/child dyad, least surprisingly because mothers are more often the ones most involved with early direct care, professional attempts at interventions, safeguarding networks, and, ultimately, court proceedings. While there is an increasing interest by researchers, practitioners, and policymakers to appreciate the seeds of vulnerability, particularly those linked to maternal functions, I am more likely to hear or read a restricted narrative about fathers and the information is often skimpy pictures titled domestic violence, coercive control, incest, or abandonment. There is rarely a multi-dimensional picture in the narratives about the father-child relationship or the nature of the mother-father couple. It is, therefore, more difficult to grapple with the complex unconscious template of fathers and couples that inhabit these young people's minds. Yet it has become difficult to enter this territory without getting tangled in the social, political, and theoretical discourses around gender and the toxic and polarising impact they can have on team discussions often resulting in defensive retreat from talking about fathers. I do not seek to resolve those issues, or to introduce new theoretical territory. Rather, it is an invitation to the reader to think about fathering, and its role in the development of an internal world, as a jigsaw piece in the complex puzzle these young people present. Furthermore, there is rarely detail about the emotional landscape of fathers, or the ghosts in their nurseries, and the language to describe them is most often behavioural rather than psychological. Many of these young people have question marks in their genograms

DOI: 10.4324/9781003020370-7

where fathers are concerned and this diagrammatic square gets filled in with idealisation or denigration, but more often with confusion.

There are two significant parenting functions in the early life of babies, which are both necessary for the healthy development of psychic functioning. The first, which has been referred to in theoretical terms as the maternal function, describes the capacity to attune to, contain, and transform the extremes of infantile emotional states, an empathic function; while the second, referred to as the paternal function, combines 'two almost conflicting functions: the *protective function* and the *prohibitive function*'. An important aspect of the paternal function is facilitating connection with and adjustment to the demands of the external world (Jung 1938, 1953 in Stevens, 1999).

In most societies, largely because of the gendered organisation of labour and home life, fathers have an instrumental role acting as the bridge between family life and the life of society at large in contrast with the mother's more expressive and caring role, concerned with the home and family. Stevens (1986) suggests that the father's role is concerned with the tangible world in the context of space and time; in other words, those aspects, which are approached, managed, and modified through consciousness and the use of one's will. In this way, a fathering role can model and encourage the development of skills necessary for successful adult adaptation to the external, social, and physical world, including the world of social relationships, work, money, politics, and power. This idea of the paternal function may be seen as the predisposition or unconscious foundation for developing the skills to deal with this 'external' world (Stevens 1986). As our society changes, the person contributing to the development of the paternal function is not always the same as the father. For the purpose of this chapter, I will, for the most part, be referring to the paternal function rather than the actual father.

However, as this is a book about child sexual exploitation, I think that the gender and relationship of the actual father in the real world, does bear some significance. The actual pathological father (or other adult male) imposes a sexual meaning on to the child's ordinary need for physical closeness and affection, thus conflating the two. In cases of incest or sexual abuse, he invites the child into assuming the role of the spouse or partner. This confusion can then become lodged in the mind of the child and disturbs later adult relationships. These adolescents, in seeking physical comfort, closeness or affection, or grappling with the ordinary challenges of establishing sexual relationships, merge these.

While early theorist developed their ideas in the context of the society they saw around them where roles were traditionally gendered, they were more significantly establishing the idea of a paternal function – in other words, the idea that one of the parents (historically the father) acts as 'a third' who, by mediating the initial symbiotic relationship between the mother and the baby, enables the beginning of the separation process for the child and encourages an entry into the social and emotional relationships of others. The father is, therefore, more than a mere rival with whom the child competes with for the mother's love, but is also the representative of the social world including the rules which govern a functioning community, society, or the wider world thus extending relationships beyond the cocoon of initial infant/mother experience. As such, it is only by establishing an identification with this paternal function that the child develops the internal scaffolding that enables it to function successfully in managing the external world. It is useful to consider how the absence of a paternal functionary or the presence of one who distorts or perverts the protective or prohibitive functions contributes to the vulnerability to sexual exploitation in these young people.

The role of this person, usually but not necessarily the partner of the primary carer, is also to support, protect, and contain the primary carer who, while in this earliest more symbiotic and permeable emotional state is more emotionally exposed. This emersion with the baby tends towards a more inward rather than outward looking state of mind and receptivity to the babies' emotional communications. A paternal functionary helps to re-establish and reconnect them to their emotional and social relationships with others besides the infant. The mother can then in time reconnect to this paternal function, which as part of her early development, she has internalised in her own mind and has drawn on to help provide a containing experience for the baby. In relation to the mother-infant dyad, the father is 'someone else' who thinks about and gets involved with the child.

As long as both of these mental functions, maternal/paternal, structure, and emotion, are benignly available, ordinary development proceeds. I would suggest that the absence or distortion of these functions or how they relate to each other might lie at the heart of vulnerability. It is this mental couple, the complementary link between emotion and structure, that establishes thinking capacity and, therefore, assists the healthy development of the child. Held within a thinking parental couple, the baby establishes its sense of self and internalises the ability to manage itself and keep itself safe. This functional partnership also enables the establishment of a psychic template about triangular relationships, self in relationship to the couple rather than the binary one of self and other – often shorthanded by attachment theory – that is relevant to working with child sexual exploitation.

It is the absence of a functioning father in this internal thinking, creative and loving couple, that might help to explain some of the difficult and often unsatisfactory relationships they make, both with predators, and with the professionals who work with them. These young people are always in action rather than reflection. While this is not uncommon in adolescents more generally, others have the capacity when alongside a containing and thoughtful adult to think about their actions, whereas these vulnerable adolescents seem to remain in action, often aggressive or risky action and cannot easily use, or actively reject the thinking mind of a helpful adult. This attack on thinking and reflection can get powerfully projected into those working with them. This may throw some light on the difficulties observed in building helpful therapeutic relationships and why teams and networks seem to have difficulties working together.

I was myself struck by how difficult it has been for me when writing about these young women with traumatic lives to keep a coherent thread or to bring structure to their complex and confusing stories. It was as if my own mind had no structure or form. It was suggested to me that it was as if in projective identification with the case material my mind had no paternal function. This loss of a capacity to think straight often permeates the experience of young people and radiates out to those working with them.

To protect anonymity, no persons or situations depicted in these next illustrations are real. They are amalgams created from aspects of people I have worked with over the years and are intended to convey the complex realities of this work. However I hope that anyone working with this population will feel that they accurately reflect the people or situations that they know.

All these young people raised concerns for professionals about Child Sexual Exploitation, and the mandatory risk assessment and forms necessary for compliance with regulatory agencies and legal frameworks were diligently completed. There might also be referral forms or extensive documentation. But often, only the sketchiest information about the father was available or perhaps even unknown. There was rarely a comment about what it had been like for the social worker to encounter these fathers, perhaps the trepidation or fear of doing a home visit while they were there. There was little mention of efforts to connect to absent father in any way. If it was there at all, it was the experience of working with the mother that was described.

I hope to illustrate by presenting these complex and difficult to work with young women more fully described below, how important it is to remember that there is a father in these stories and how their behaviours may, in part, be connected to the disturbed parental functions and distorted triangular relationships that inhabit their minds, unconsciously as well as consciously.

It is important to remember that CSE is not a one-off meeting, like stranger rape or the powerlessness of a dependent child on an abusing parent. Groomers may have undergone a similar dysfunctional relationship to their victims. It is the unconscious re-creation of earlier dysfunctional relationships, where the groomers' social and psychological pathology fit with the couple relationships these vulnerable young people retain as unconscious templates in their minds. Stories told by and about these young people are often about meeting with groomers again and again, feeling like they are in desired relationships with them, feeling special at least to start with, and often including a perverse sense of being the one in control. It can also lead to dynamics of blame, denigration, exclusion, or powerlessness, which can be projected into or between the workforces charged with protecting and caring for them.

Anna

When Anna was little, her father would often come home drunk. His lyrical singing, loud humour, and demanding presence would quickly escalate into abusive and cruel words and, often, physical assault. Anna's mother would pick baby Anna up in a rough attempt at protection and put her in the bedroom, shushing her in words she couldn't have understood, entreating her not to make a sound but not containing her fears. Anna would lie on the bed with noise wafting through, frozen in fear until she fell asleep. She would often wake to a crying mother and snoring father.

Anna inevitably witnessed a great deal of domestic violence early in her life. She had to manage her terror and the fear and abandonment cycle on her own, often falling asleep to block out the sounds and feelings of the abusive environment.

One note in the file's chronology described her as a toddler who laughed when she was with her father, and she was often seen 'holding his hand'. Yet records show that she had been seen in A&E twice with a sprain and bruising when she was a toddler, after being alone in her father's care. At six, on the at-risk register, she moved to her grandmother's care, but grandmother was frightened of her daughter and son-in-law and returned her at their insistence. At seven, she came to school with bruising and told her teacher that her father had hit her.

She was placed on a care order and after a temporary foster placement where she settled quickly, she was moved to a long-term foster placement with a single foster mother. She moved without protest but found it hard to settle and continued to have sleep disturbances. Supervised contact with her mother continued, but as her mother seemed unable to separate from her partner, and sometimes arrived at contact smelling of alcohol, this contact was restricted. After being assessed, Anna was diagnosed with early relational trauma. She lived with Ms S for almost seven years, but Ms S said that Anna's behaviour was getting out of control and felt she could no longer cope with her. She worried that Anna was hanging around with older boys, who have all been excluded from school but seem to have lots of money and give her gifts. Anna says she hates school and frequently refuses to attend, she won't see her social worker except to demand more money and says her foster mother is being unreasonable about her rules and wants her to leave her alone. She taunted the foster carer saying that she was single because nobody loved her and had started to steal from her, and the foster carer found alcohol in her bedroom. When the placement broke down, she was placed in a small residential unit for adolescents.

Anna wanted to be called AJ. She didn't want a girl's name as girls were useless.

At the beginning, she was charming, engaging with staff, and saying how much better this placement was than living with her foster carer. The staff, however, felt they were walking on eggshells with her and that any refusal to provide whatever she wanted would meet with an explosive barrage of verbal abuse and threats of violence. During a consultation, they joked it was like living with Jekyll and Hyde but were stunned by the link I drew to the description of her father in her early years. When she started staying out past curfews and returning drunk and unkempt, the staff became concerned about whether she was involved with sexual predators.

When they tried to talk to her about it, she told them to 'fuck off' and leave her alone. She began to mock staff for their uselessness, and play one off against the other, as if proving that they did not communicate. Her 'favourite' staff member fluctuated, often being experienced by the staff as her wanting to 'get them on side'. Despite discussion of this at staff meetings, it seemed difficult to remember in the moment, and their interactions with her, and often the responses of agency cover staff, was to be pulled unconsciously into those scripts. The police became involved as concerns grew that she was being pulled into sex trafficking. As her contact with the gang of men increased her behaviour at the home became more aggressive, threatening, and unreasonable.

The father in Anna's mind was unpredictable and shifted between the lyrical and playful and the dangerous and cruel. She desired one and feared awakening the other. The protective aspect of the paternal function was perverted into riskiness since the capacity for benign firmness, the cornerstone of a healthy parent in mind, had not been internalised. For Anna, this gang of men and their tricky girlfriends had a repetitive pull. Being drawn to the attention they bestowed on her, their singing rap lyrics for her, the coercive control over her clothes and hairstyle, and provision of drink – which all put her at odds with the staff – contained an unconscious echo of her father returning home from drinking with his mates. And the same humour and intrusive presence would quickly become demanding and then escalate into abusive and cruel words and, often, physical assault. Returned by the police after being reported missing again and again, bruised, sexually assaulted, and drunk, it made it difficult for professionals to understand why she kept returning to these abusers.

Like her mother who was only allowed limited contact with her, her desire for connection to these men was stronger than her capacity for separation. Her internal couple was one where coercive control was a dominant feature.

The abusers, like fathers, needed to be placated. Their gifts and praise unpredictably transformed into exclusion or cruelty. Anna's infant childhood experience of safety was the denial and shutting down of her infancy. 'Fingers in ears' became drink and drugs and the refusal to believe or trust those who claimed they would keep her safe. In denigrating and belittling the ineffectual staff and seeking out the cruel and perverse, Anna was communicating how, in her mind, there was no benign mental couple providing a link between emotion and structure. The baby Anna had never established an internal capacity to manage herself and keep herself safe. The staff team became ineffectual and the abusive men she was drawn towards were, in her mind, the ones that she needed to attend to.

Without an experience of a benign couple, safety was also an unconscious identification with the aggressor. Frankel (2002) describes how identification with the aggressor can be connected to responses to trauma, emotional abandonment, or powerlessness. Over time, it can become habitual and can lead to cruelty, aggression, hyper vigilance, and distortions in reality testing. I think it is helpful to think about it as a possible response to early trauma when there is a defensive disconnection of affect from experience. You remember the abuse but not the feelings of powerlessness, rage, or fear.

Anna was bullying and controlling with staff. By internalising the behaviour of the aggressor, in this case, Anna's father, the 'victim' hopes (unconsciously) to avoid abuse and may begin to feel an emotional connection with the abuser, which distorts feelings of empathy. Identification with the aggressor is a version of introjection that focuses on the adoption, not of general or positive traits, but of negative or feared traits. If you are afraid of someone, you can unconsciously partially conquer that fear by becoming more like them.

There is more of a pull towards an unconscious familiarity with something in these perpetrators than to the unfamiliar unconscious scripts of caring, helpful, curious, and reflective professionals. It is not to say that the external realities of money, gifts, and pleasure are not part of what draws those in poverty, deprivation, despair, or depression to join gangs or stay with the groomers. But the unconscious compulsion to recreate earlier relational templates is more powerful because there has been no early containment, the mind, and availability of another who helps process the trauma.

Freud (1922) first established the idea of 'repetition compulsion' when he described how a patient does not always remember things but instead seems to act them out without knowing that he is repeating it. We might recognise this if we've met women who with help have extricated themselves at great personal cost and with relief from situations of domestic violence, including being settled in new accommodation, only to form relationships with new partners where abuse or coercive control surface. Change is not only dealing with the external realities such as new homes or finances but also a professional relationship that enables thinking about the phenomenon.

According to this idea, there are two ways to process the past. Either through reflective thinking, which creates memory, or through 'repetition compulsion', which is the unconscious phenomenon of putting oneself in the same situation again and again. In repetition compulsion, we keep recreating early relationships because they have not been processed into memory. Instead, we return to them in the hope that it will be different. But in order for that to happen, you have to 'properly remember, think about and feel what happened to you. And who can blame you for avoiding this?' (Stubley 2023).

Repetitions of traumatic events can be for the purpose of achieving control over its outcome. Like with toddlers who repeat games again and again, the repetition is a move towards mastery. A victim of sexual abuse or incest may later participate in abusive or exploitative relationships with a view to finding a different outcome.

The pull to repeat is very powerful. So advice or sympathy alone, however well intended, can't always reach these ghosts from the past. Anna's pull towards groomers and denigration of those struggling to provide helpful care was a recreation of the internal triangle she had absorbed from her earliest years. The bonhomie of the initial contact with these men, which turned unpredictably to a cruel exploitation, had an unremembered echo of her birth father. And in the attempt at gathering her up and metaphorically putting her in her room to keep her safe from exploitation, the residential staff became the ineffectual protector of her childhood.

Anna never talked about her father and declared she could not remember him when the social worker worked on a genogram. She laughed scornfully at any suggestion that the men she was with were like her dad. Attempts at talking with her 'logically' or offering advice became frustrating, even infuriating for some professionals, because it was met with the absence of thinking space in her mind.

Barbara

Barbara's father left before she was born. Barbara was born to a 19-year-old mother, Dee, who already had one child living with her mother. Dee struggled with what had been diagnosed as a bipolar disorder and used alcohol as a means to anesthetise herself from the hurt and rejection of multiple partners who 'loved me and left me'. Her mother told her that her father had abandoned them both and run off with another woman. She refused to discuss him saying they were safer without him. There was a suggestion that he had been part of a gang involved with drugs. Records suggest he had been sent to prison for a serious drug trafficking offence.

Her mother struggled to raise Barbara and two subsequent children who all moved between a single maternal grandmother, a single aunt, and time with her. By the age of ten, Barbara was being described as 'out of control' and too aggressive towards her younger siblings.

At 12, Barbara started cutting herself as she had read on social media that it was a way to manage her depression, and at 13, she was near to being excluded from school and concerns were raised about the 'gang' of kids she was on the periphery of. Barbara was referred for a residential placement at age 14. Despite attempts around formalising Special Guardianship orders with her maternal grandmother and a paternal aunt, both quickly 'returned' her.

After telling a teacher she had been drunk and had sex with one of the older boys, there were finally court proceedings, and Barbara was put in Care. First placed in foster care, she threatened the carers' daughter and stole things from her. Her behaviour grew increasingly sexualised, and the foster father felt anxious if he was in a room with her alone. When that placement was terminated, she was deemed too challenging for a foster placement and was found a place in a small residential unit for adolescents.

At staff meetings, there were secretive feelings expressed about not wanting to spend time with her. They observed some staff members would choose the activities that she was least likely to be involved in or take a different resident shopping so they would not be available to take her to the gym. She actively sought out the attention of a senior male member of staff, Joe. In the living room, she would try to sit between him and the other resident or staff he was sitting next to as the group of residents watched TV, and sat next to him at meals.

Anyone who has spent time in the company of a young child recognises the tragic comedy of the toddler squeezing themselves between the parents who are sitting closely together. But who hasn't witnessed the agony when the toddler watched their carer talking to another and tries to grab their face and turn it towards themselves or pull at the clothes or in an unbearable moment, slap the adult, to reclaim the attention towards themselves. To carefully observe the child, one must bear the desperation of having to share the precious attentiveness towards them with another. The parental management of this experience for the child is fundamental for ordinary development and future emotional well-being. The degree to which the need to intrude, grab, or push into that couple, or manage the loneliness of feeling excluded again, becomes established as an unconscious view of relationships. For Barbara, this was not managed helpfully in her early experience.

On a consultation visit to meet with the staff team, I walked past Barbara and noted that she was right up and in the face of a staff member demanding her pocket money. That staff member looked over at me as I passed and said hello. Barbara moved slightly to block me out of the line of vision. She blanked me and then told me to 'fuck off and mind my own business'. As I walked out towards the meeting room she said loudly, 'why is that Bitch staring at me'?

This 'third position' (Britton 1989) explains how initially the child develops a capacity to be a participant in a relationship and observed by a third and be an observer of a relationship between two people. This sets the foundation for thinking and reflection. The problem for the team was that Barbara would refuse to join activities with other staff. She always appeared to like whatever it was that Joe was about to take other residents to do. When she was with Joe, other staff members described feeling unwanted and un-needed. They would often retreat into the office to do their paperwork. She complained that the staff did not like her. There were several incidents when she would damage the office door in her attempts to speak to staff that were inside. The staff team had various disagreements about how to work with her and some became quite judgemental about or angry with Joe.

One Saturday, Barbara cut her arm after being ghosted by classmates on their WhatsApp Group. Joe, the only one with a driving license on shift, took her to A&E. After triage, they were asked to wait and spent a long time in a crowded waiting area. Barbara kept leaning on Joe, trying to stroke his hair, and giggling loudly. He asked her to stop on numerous occasions, to which she replied she didn't feel well and might faint. At one point, the nurse in charge approached him and, on taking him aside, said there had been a series of 'concerned complaints' about them by other patients. Joe quickly phoned a female colleague who came to join them. He had to stay, as he had the car, but moved to a seat a few rows behind them in the waiting area. Barbara sat a seat away from the female staff member mumbling about why she had to come and didn't they trust Joe to stay with her. I had found Joe in staff meetings to be a responsible thoughtful man. The manager confirmed his ability to maintain professional boundaries. He found Barbara's limpet like and seductive approaches disturbing, and found the only way to keep appropriate distance was to withdraw from contact with her.

For Barbara, there had not been a helpful internalisation of a 'third'. There were only couples. This was true of her time with her grandmother and her aunt. Separation in these couple was dependent on actual rending them asunder – sending them into care. She could find no comfortable place alongside an adult couple. Wedging herself between the foster carers or residential workers, and in competition with other siblings and residents, she could only relate as a couple. Her fixation on an exclusive relationship with an idealised male staff member seemed to be recreated later when Barbara became fixated on an older man who had been buying her gifts. It took many months and police involvement to charge this man with grooming and sexual assault. For Barbara, without a father in the real world, but also, importantly, without anyone who had provided a helpful paternal function, she idealised the absent parent causing a distortion of reality. In the absence of the father, some children might substitute an exotic or romanticised other, the equivalent of

Tracy Beaker's mother, or a prince charming who is off on adventures but will return to rescue the child from their current circumstances.

Barbara's father in mind was an idealised absent father. In her mind, he was taken from her against his will, and any information in her files that said that he had been contacted many times to enable contact between them was said by her to be a lie. Her denial of his abandonment, re-enforced by the abandonment of other adults with parenting tasks, was so profound, that despite reality testing, she continued to maintain the idea that he had been trying for many years to find her. Her seductive demeanour and desire to connect to an absent father were recreated in the relationships she tried to form with men. It might help us to understand more the nature of the pull towards groomers who, with their gifts and compliments, create a caricature of the idealised father, the father who wanted her and stayed. She had a lack of a protective or prohibitive father in mind.

Carmel

Carmel's father 'chose her' when she was prepubescent. He had come and gone in her life, often arriving with gifts and treats but then leaving again with no warning. He said her mother was 'spoiled goods', someone who was up to no good when he was not around, but that she was his beautiful, pure darling, her daddy's princess. On occasion, she was allowed to stay at his house. She loved being his 'special girl' but felt worried when he would climb into bed with her smelling like beer. Her older sister had left home pregnant a few years earlier, and her younger brother was still treated like a baby. He had a different dad, who paid very little attention to Carmel.

Carmel came to the attention of social services when the school noticed she was cutting and made a referral. She often appeared distracted, and despite being a bright young woman, she was falling very far behind in her schoolwork. Carmel started cutting herself as she had read on social media that it made you feel no pain. Then she started coming to school smelling of cannabis and lurking near the school gates with a much older man. Her attitude became more oppositional and aggressive. After a series of further self-harm/suicidal incidents, she was briefly hospitalised, and upon discharge, she was taken into care and placed in a small residential unit. She was said to have problems with peer relationships. She decried any rules of the children's home as institutionalised and babyish. She refused to participate in any of the activities designed for the residents. The other female residents were either afraid of her or desperate to befriend her. She would hang around with a male resident with reported links to drugs and county lines. She often left the home very late and, after being reported missing, returned in the early hours of the morning with new phone or clothes and, when asked about them, said they were things she bought from money her father, who she was not allowed to have contact with, had put in her account.

Stocky in build 14-year-old Carmel would take up a pugilistic bodily stance and talk loud and fast and over other people's words preventing any actual discussion or exchange. Her moods and behaviour moved between high dependency, demanding relationships, and serious aggression directed at any sign of a staff member not complying with her demands. Following these confrontations, she would often run away. Her volatility made staff anxious and described having to walk on eggshells so as not to trigger an aggressive response – either towards a person or property – actually hurting staff members and trashing communal space. The staff found her neediness exhausting and her changing state of mind confusing. They felt she was always testing boundaries and playing one staff member off against another. Her running away was becoming more regular, and the very caring staff regularly had to report her missing to the police. On her return, she would often have jewellery or consumer items, which she called gifts, and flared up when the staff tried to discuss whom she had been with or what she had been doing. Although the staff worked extremely hard to engage with her and diligently checked her phone and online accounts, they remained concerned that they could not keep her safe. The network was extremely concerned about her being used for sex work.

New to care work, Peter, a graduate who was finding his city job uninspiring, brought a genuine desire to help these young people. His friendly and handsome demeanour and similar cultural profile made him the staff member Carmel most often searched out. Peter was friendly and had some similar interests in music. He would share stories of his own life in an attempt to make a connection. Having not realised why, when in his initial training he was advised not to use social media without caution, he had put personal photos on his Instagram feed. Some included his girlfriend. His manager, alert to Carmel's demanding and intrusive manner with him, discussed the issue of boundaries in their supervision and suggested he keep a more distant, less befriending position. In a concrete attempt to do as was suggested, he reiterated that he was staff, and told Carmel that there needed to be firmer boundaries and they weren't friends. She retorted by saying she never wanted to be friends with him, he was as old as her father, and stormed away. Later that day, she made an allegation that he was putting the moves on her, and that he had porn on his phone. She said that he had also assaulted another young person in the home.

Of course, the proper protocols were immediately put in place, and a referral made to the Local Authority Designated Officer[1] who is responsible for coordinating the response to concerns that an adult who works with children may have caused them or could cause them harm.

Peter was suspended pending an investigation. As per the requirements, an independent practitioner interviewed all his colleagues, managers, and young people. New to the work, he was angry about Carmel's lies, and his family was worried for the impact on his life and career. Having never been alone on shift with Carmel, his colleagues were able to attest to the unsubstantiated nature of the allegations, and the other young people also said that they had not made allegations and Peter had done nothing to them. They said that Carmel had bragged to them that 'staff always do what she wants or else'. After a thorough investigation, there were no concerns about his actual behaviours. But Peter was left bruised by the allegations and fearful about future working. Carmel trashed her bedroom and attacked a staff member who had become angry with Carmel about her 'lies' about Peter. Her placement was put seriously at risk, and she absconded and was found a few days later at the home of an older man with whom she had engaged in sexual activity. It was evident that they had been drinking and using drugs. When this was described as abuse, she insisted that she had instigated it and she wasn't a victim.

Her complaint against Peter seemed to stem from a grievance. Grievances can act as a container for everything negative. While grief may lead to mourning and emergence from loss, grievance, especially stemming from early parental loss, may lead to the frozen, deadened preoccupation with what has been lost. To develop, one has to grieve the loss of the good experience, to grieve for what was not available or what you can't have. For Carmel, she must grieve never having had an ordinary relationship with her father. Without this, grief can get stuck as grievance and prevent the use of the availability of those trying to provide help. For staff there can be a risk that some young people make repeated complaints. The novice care worker who at first was trying to relate in a friendly manner but who following supervision, rigidly withdrew, stirred up Carmel's confusion over generational boundaries and roles. In her internal world, you were either inappropriately inside or outside the couple. There was no possible safe third position. Peter was either a sexual partner or gotten rid of. His unexplained abandonment, first through withdrawing his 'friendship' and then by his immediate required suspension, confirmed her expectation.

The helpful father in mind is one who establishes a protective and prohibitive internal scaffold. For Carmel, childhood incest and domestic violence distorted and perverted these functions. These, in turn, perverted her relationships.

Harding (2001, cited in Wood, 2003), presents a contemporary description of what is meant by perversity, considering not whether sexuality or types of sexual behaviour is normal or perverse but whether it is used expressively or defensively. Sex used to enhance intimacy and the sense of self and others is different from its use to protect the self or others from anxiety, or to disguise or erotise aggression and hostility. In other words, it is not what 'type' of sex but rather what feelings are being expressed and what is being communicated through the sexual encounters. One indicator of perversity in this framework she suggests, is the rapid oscillations between victim and perpetrator (Wood 2003).

For young women like Carmel, not only is there a dysfunctional couple in mind, but often one where there is a couple whose relationship is perverse. Incest for Carmel was a sexual relation with her father from which her mother was excluded and denigrated. Generational boundaries were blurred. Many young women who are vulnerable as a result of earlier abuse can become easily targeted. The dysfunctional paternal or inadequate maternal objects in their emotional landscapes fit with the needs and pathology of the predators. Attempts to dissuade or prevent these relationships are met with incredulity by the young women who state categorically that it is their choice and their decision. Social workers, residential workers, and others in these young people's professional networks are required under Section 1 of the Children Act 1989, 'to take account of the ascertainable wishes and feelings of the child concerned considered in the light of his age and understanding' (Gov.uk 1989). Yet to "ascertain" wishes and feelings of the young person without a way to think about these unconscious dynamics, might get confused with believing they cannot object to the young person's "lifestyle choice". Sometimes also, the confusion of generational boundaries gets played out in this domain of "choice"; the young person who challenges objections by asking "what is wrong with me dating older men?". Often, drugs and alcohol are part of the exploitation. But like the narcotic effect of other addictions, sexual exploitation hooks into the distortions established through the violent or abusive sexual connections of the couples in mind. A perverse aspect of child sexual exploitation is how often these young women describe themselves as being in control or having the power. In this way, sexual behaviour can be used unconsciously as a means of self-expression, self-protection, or self-destructiveness (ibid). Unlike other high-risk behaviours or destructive addictions, sexual exploitation has until recently, been described as a conscious choice rather than a serious psychological disturbance.

Staff employed in caring for adolescents have their own fathers in mind. Some may have been absent, authoritarian, or idealised. It is not a requirement for residential staff to have been in therapy or discuss their own early experiences. A supervisor or consultant's interest in their early lives is often experienced as intrusive or unnecessary. Yet without reflection, the ghosts of their own fathers may haunt their work. It may make it more difficult not to get drawn into the unconscious scripts of the residents when living in such a family like environment for extended periods of time. And it may make it more difficult to bring fathering into discussions with and about the young people.

While exploring sexual relationships is part of ordinary adolescent development, those most vulnerable to sexual exploitation often have 'couples in mind' where coercive control, narcissism, abandonment, cruelty, fear, and denigration have taken the place of the more ordinary internalised parents who offer a template of supportive, loving, and creative coupling. In ordinary relationships, physicality is benign, and thinking can happen. The sex, in sexual exploitation, can be more about the distorted meaning of bodily contact not actually a mutually satisfying sexual exchange. For the young vulnerable women where the paternal function of support, protection, prohibition, and establishing a third position has not been internalised and there is no safe mental couple, the complementary link between emotion and regulation which forms the capacity for thinking and acting safely in the world, is diminished. This leads to action and not thought, exploitation and not mutuality. For those working in close proximity to those young people, they can get caught up in this as well. To grapple with Child Sexual Exploitation, workers need to consider how the exploitative and dysfunction dynamics of these internal worlds get transposed into relationships in the world outside.

Note

1 The role of the Local Authority Designated Officer, LADO, is set out in chapter 2 of the HM Government Guidance Working Together to Safeguard Children (July 2018) the London Child Protection Procedures (Chapter 7, 6th Edition 2017), DfE Keeping Children Safe in Education (September 2019).

References

Britton, R. (1989) *The missing link: parental sexuality in the Oedipal complex*, in Steiner, J. Britton,R. et al (eds) (1989), Abingdon, oxford: Routledge.

Davies, N. and Eagle, G. (2013) Contemporary Psychoanalysis, 49 (4) p 559, 27p (function 2).

Frankel, J. (2002) *Exploring Ferenczi's concept of identification with the aggressor: It's role in trauma, everyday life and therapeutic relationships.* Psychoanalytic Dialogues, 12(1), pp. 101–139.

Freud, S. (1922) *Beyond the Pleasure Principle, The Standard Edition of the complete psychological works of Sigmund Freud*, 180:1–283, London, The Hogarth Press.

Gov.uk (1989) *The Children Act 1989 guidance and regulations.* https://assets.publishing.service.gov.uk/government/uploads/system/uploads/attachment_data/file/1000549/The_Children_Act_1989_guidance_and_regulations_Volume_2_care_planning__placement_and_case_review.pdf

Stevens, A. (1986) *The Father: Contemporary Jungian Perspectives.* London, Free Association Books.

Stevens, A. (1999) *On Jung.* New Jersey, Princeton University Press.

Stubley, J. In *Ask Annalisa Barbieri* (2023, May 12). www.theguardian.com

Wood, H. (2003) *Psychoanalytic theories of perversion reformulated.* Reformulation, Summer, pp. 26–31.

8

THE SOCIAL AND POLITICAL CONTEXT

Steve Bambrough and R.M. Shingleton

In this chapter, we would like to explore some of the legislative and social policy context in the UK relating to child sexual abuse and exploitation, how effective this framework is, and what conclusions we can draw from this.

The National Society for the Prevention of Cruelty to children (NSPCC) estimates in their prevalence study that roughly 1 in 20 11–17-year-olds in England and Wales have experienced contact abuse in relation to sexual abuse (NSPCC 2021). A Home Office report (Home Office 2017) estimates that only 10% of children and young people reported this to someone "in an official position" then the scale of the problem is significant. In the United States, it is estimated that 10% of children aged 0–17 have been exposed to sexual abuse and other forms of sexual harm (Letourneau et al. 2014). In 2020, the Office for National Statistics (Office of National Statistics 2020) estimated that there are 3.1 million adults in England and Wales who had experienced sexual abuse by the age of 16. It is, therefore, not surprising that the WHO has identified child sexual abuse as one of the 24 global public health problems (Mathers, Stevens, Mascarenhas 2009).

Although child sexual exploitation (CSE) does not have a legislative definition in English law, nor is it a specific criminal offence in itself, it is recognised within safeguarding and criminal justice and there is a substantial amount of legislation that can be used to address it. Within safeguarding, public law proceedings including the use of Secure Accommodation Orders (S.25 of the Children Act 1989) and regulations such as the Children (Secure Accommodation) Regulations 1991 can be effective in finding a safe environment and support for a child or young person.

Recovery Orders can be sought by a local authority when a child or young person who is being sexually exploited is in care. Civil injunctions against

DOI: 10.4324/9781003020370-8

perpetrators under the Inherent Jurisdiction have also been used when the aim is to regulate the conduct of those who have been proven to be perpetrators. Where a child or young person is the subject of CSE, then it may be appropriate for the local authority to share parental responsibility under an interim or final care order under the 1989 Act. However, this potential remedy exposes one of the serious complications about CSE in relation to the 1989 Act – that is, the parent/s are often *not* the source of the risk of sexual exploitation (PACE 2019).

In English criminal law, there is no specific offence of CSE and the harmful behaviour in question will be treated as falling within the relevant sexual offence under the Sexual Offences Act 2003. Prior to this Act, the Sexual Offences Act 1956 was the primary piece of legislation covering sexual offending. The sexual offences covered in the 2003 Act include rape, sexual assault, sexual offences against children under 13 (s. 5–8), and sexual activity with a child (ss 9–13). S.14 of this Act creates an offence of arranging or facilitating a child sexual offence.

Statutory guidance published as "Safeguarding children involved in prostitution" (DoH 2000) made it clear to health, police, and social services that this was exploitation. This guidance was added to in 2003 by the Sexual Offences Act which made it an offence to arrange or facilitate child pornography or pay for sexual acts with a child or arrange or facilitate the sexual exploitation of a child.

Several further updates to law and guidance such as (in Scotland) the Protection of Children and Prevention of Sexual Offences (Scotland) Act 2005 make it a statutory offence to meet a child for sexual purposes.

Previous to this, in 1996, Britain adopted the Stockholm Declaration at the First World Congress against the Commercial Sexual Exploitation of Children, which declared that this was "a form of coercion and violence against children" (Stockholm Declaration 1996) – a definition which would be useful to have been born in mind during the years of sexual exploitation of children and young people abuse which has been exposed by numerous reviews, inquiries, and investigations.

In England, there is an expectation that people working with children will comply with the key statutory guidance for child protection, *Working Together to Safeguard Children* (Department for Education July 2022) which was updated most recently in 2022. This stipulates that everyone who works with children has a responsibility for keeping them safe, and every individual who comes into contact with children and families has a role to play in sharing information and identifying concerns.

In Wales, the key guidance is *Working Together to Safeguard People* and is based on the requirements set out in the Social Services and Well-being (Wales) Act 2014, supported by the *Wales Safeguarding Procedures*. It is mainly aimed at practitioners working with children, including early years, social care, education, health, the police, youth offending and youth, community, and family support services (including the third sector) and foster care and residential care. This sets out detailed practice guidance expectations about how individuals and organisations will work together in safeguarding children.

So, through a combination of legislation (the Serious Crime Act 2015; Sexual Offences Act 2003; Justice Act (Northern Ireland) 2015; Sexual Offences (Northern Ireland) Order 2008; Sexual Offences (Scotland) Act 2009; Protection of Children and Prevention of Sexual Offences (Scotland) Act 2005) in the United Kingdom it is illegal to:

- cause or incite a child to engage in sexual activity
- meet a child following sexual grooming
- have sexual communication with a child
- take, make, or have indecent photographs of children
- sexually exploit a child (including paying for or arranging sexual services of a child)

This suggests that the legislation exists in the United Kingdom for the appropriate protection of children and young people from sexual exploitation, but how effective is it in practice?

Given the failings of statutory bodies to protect children and young people from sexual exploitation in several high-profile cases during the last three decades, there has been a great deal of subsequent focus on social policy. A Barnardo's report (Barnardo's 2014) of the parliamentary inquiry into the effectiveness of legislation for tackling CSE and trafficking in the United Kingdom chaired by Sarah Champion MP, concluded that the legislation is "generally sound", but the inquiry found consistent concerns about how the legislation was *understood and applied*.

Detective Superintendent Ian Critchley, Lancashire Constabulary, is quoted in this report as saying that the legislation "is good enough and largely appropriate". A young person giving evidence to the inquiry more graphically said, "I looked up the Sexual Offences Act last night and it looks like a good law. It's the fact that the police don't care, and social workers have too many cases and sexual health services don't know what to do".

The Inspector of Constabulary, in the introduction to The National Child Protection Inspections (2019) thematic report (the first being in 2015), said that "much more needed to be done to ensure that all children in need of help and protection received the right help at the right time" and that a "new model is required that considers the root causes of vulnerability and takes steps to address them. New statutory Safeguarding partnerships (underpinned by legislation) represent such an opportunity" (National Child Protection Inspections 2019). This reference to the safeguarding partnerships was a significant change introduced by the Children and Social Work Act 2017, which replaced Local Safeguarding Children Boards (LSCBs) with local safeguarding arrangements led by three safeguarding partners (local authorities, chief officers of police, and clinical commissioning groups).

Sarah Nelson, in her excellent book *Tackling Child Sexual Abuse* (Nelson 2016), writes that the point in describing already existing law, guidance, and social policy such as we have tried to do here is;

> to emphasise how clear these were. Yet they continued to be widely flouted and ignored by key protective agencies nearly two decades later. We have to ask why?… those of us who have campaigned for decades against CSA have been pressing many of the same arguments for 20 or 30 years.
>
> *(p. 138)*

This point is made often in the recent literature on CSE. Alexis Jay's (2014) report as part of the independent enquiry into CSE in Rotherham, made the point that:

> The police had excellent procedures from 1998, but in practice these appear to have been widely disregarded …. children as young as 11 were deemed to be having consensual sexual intercourse when in fact they were being raped and abused by adults.
>
> *(Jay 2014, p. 69; Gladman and Heal 2017, p. 55)*

The independent inquiry into child sexual abuse

This theme was further explored in "The Independent Inquiry into Child Sexual Abuse" report by Alexis Jay amongst others (Jay 2022). Its report, released in October 2022 after seven years of investigation, is a huge piece of work which sets out the extent to which state and non-state institutions failed in their duty to protect children and young people from sexual abuse and exploitation. It draws from 15 investigations, 19 related investigation reports, and 41 other Inquiry reports. It deserves much more attention than we can give it here, but we have drawn out some issues relevant to this discussion. It clearly states that:

> "The protection of personal and institutional reputations above the protection of children was a frequent institutional reaction" and the Inquiry also identified "wider societal issues where responses to children's disclosures were characterized by embarrassment, fear and disbelief". In the case of Nottingham City Council and Nottinghamshire County Council, the Inquiry found that over five decades "neither council learned from its mistakes,

despite commissioning many reviews which made it clear what changes were needed in their care systems to stop the sexual abuse of children".

It points out that there has been a recent "significant increase in child sexual exploitation online" and there is a "stark debate between protection of privacy and protection of children. A technical solution is now overdue to assist the detection of online-facilitated child sexual abuse and to make the internet safe for all children".

The Inquiry found that "despite 20 years of enhanced focus on safeguarding, schools are not as safe for children as they should be, and the children's interests do not always come first when allegations or concerns of sexual abuse arise".

The Inquiry's thematic investigation about effective leadership of child protection across its numerous investigations found that "the worst examples involved people in charge of institutions who demonstrated indifference, even hostility, to victims, despite evidence or suspicion of wrongdoing by perpetrators".

Moving onto themes of societal attitudes and terminology used in describing child sexual abuse, we can learn something from the judgemental classifications and terminology used in this area. Some services set up in the early 1990s (such as Barnardo's "Streets & Lanes" project set up in 1994 in Bradford) were aimed specifically at this group of children who were seen as being highly vulnerable to what was at that time often called "child prostitution". Sarah Swann (2000) was the manager of that project, and she could not have been clearer in her analysis that there was *no such thing as un-coerced choice* – child prostitutes did not exist but what *did* exist were abused children and child abusers. Swann's model was subsequently widely publicised through Barnardo's "Whose Daughter Next?" report as best practice.

Government statutory guidance "Safeguarding children involved in prostitution" (DoH 2000) despite its use of the term "prostitution" made it absolutely clear that this was exploitation. This shift and qualification in the use of language and terminology can be seen as a progression of the way the problem was seen "from control and punishment to care and welfare" (Melrose 2004). Melrose makes the telling point that "until relatively recently the problem of young people sexually exploited through prostitution was consistently denied … it was not a problem that practitioners and policy makers were willing to confront". Terminology such as "young sex worker" was used by some in the field but as Pitts (1997) points out, this only served to conceal the "enormity of the violation to which these young people were subject".

The DrewReview (Drew 2016) wrote that police had "too narrow a definition of child sexual exploitation" and that police attitudes and views that CSE was about "red light areas" and "gangs of men principally of Pakistani heritage" led police to look for signs of exploitation in the wrong places.

One superintendent is quoted, characterising the local problem as being "white European males, in their 40s, making extensive use of the internet for initial grooming, often of boys, and not operating as gangs at all".

The falsely held police views identified here by Professor John Drew are also reflected in mainstream media – the *Times* article (18 January 2020; "Rotherham police chief: we ignored sex abuse of children") reports a senior police officer as admitting that "his force ignored the sexual abuse of girls by Pakistani grooming gangs for decades because it was afraid of increasing 'racial tensions'".

The important issue of ethnicity in the media reporting and public perception of CSE is too large a subject to be covered in this chapter, so it is not my intention to address it here, however, we would like to raise the point made by Cockbain and Tufail (2020) that the *Sunday Times* breached reporting codes with one of its headlines which stated "Asians make up 80% of child groomers" and in doing so ignored national datasets which show that Asian men are *not* overrepresented amongst the 172,000 men convicted of sexual offences in England and Wales 2016.

Racism has also played a part in social and policing attitudes towards black children and young people. The excellent work by Jahnine Davis (2019) found in her professional practice and research that:

"Black girls were 'missing' from research, policy, and practice ...". "Problematic behaviours" related to gangs were the most frequent risk discussed; these girls seem only to be seen through this lens and are not perceived as potential victims of sexual abuse. Davis concludes that a plausible reason why Black girls may not be thought of as vulnerable to CSA is the practice of 'adultification'. Epstein, Blake, and Gonzalez (2017) found that "from the age of five, African American girls were viewed as more adult-like throughout all stages of childhood in comparison to their White peers. This increased at age 10–14 where they were perceived as more mature and sexually aware, and less innocent". Jones and Trottman's 2009 study of CSA in the Eastern Caribbean made similar findings and the phenomenon was then conceptualised as 'adultification' (Goff et al, 2014). These studies found that the general understanding of the 'normative child' – innocent, vulnerable and in need of protection – is White.

The Probation Inspectorate published Jahnine Davis' "Adultification bias within child protection and safeguarding" (Davis 2022), which highlights that "Recently, the concept of adultification bias has increasingly become a main point of discussion in child welfare arenas and the wider public space". Notable here is the case of Child Q, described by the Institute of Race Relations (John 2022) as; "state-sanctioned rape of a minor, enabled by a school which clearly abandoned its duty of care to that child. So, intent it was on criminalising her, that it was not satisfied that its own search had confirmed what she had told them, i.e., that she did not possess any cannabis. Our target must therefore be not just the police and the school, but the state which empowers both of them".

The "Child Q Local Child Safeguarding Practice Review" (City and Hackney Safeguarding Children Partnership, 2022) is one of the first reviews in England to explicitly refer to adultification as factor influencing the safeguarding of a Black child. In conclusion, Davis writes that:

> If the starting point is to question the existence of racism and racialised stereotypes, instead of how its existence can misguide child protection and safeguarding services, Black children, including those from other ethnic minority backgrounds may have their needs overlooked and erased. The adultification of Black children must be understood as a manifestation of racism. This can result in the onus of children to safeguard themselves, rather than receiving the care and protection they have a right to receive. Adultification can lead to a victim-blaming narrative, which implies Black children are somehow complicit in the harm experienced. As Black children are less likely to be afforded care, compassion, and support, it raises a serious question of who are more likely to be categorised as deserving and underserving children when in need of safeguarding and protection?

After having surveyed the very large amount of documentation covering the sexual abuse of children during the writing of this chapter, we find no reason to disagree with Angie Heal's analysis that this is the "biggest child protection scandal in UK history … The inaction and indifference by senior police officers and Rotherham Council staff to what was occurring on their watch is still difficult to comprehend despite the countless attempts by social commentators to make sense of what happened" (Gladman and Heal 2017).

Returning to the Independent Inquiry into Child Sexual Abuse, the Inquiry's analysis revealed, the issue of child sexual abuse was "concealed from public view for decades. Poor attitudes towards children compromised the ability of institutions to expose and act on allegations of child sexual abuse. There was no real understanding of the scale and depravity of that abuse until national scandals were exposed, such as the posthumous revelations made about Jimmy Savile in 2012 and the conviction in 2015 of Bishop Peter Ball. Even then, some forms of child sexual exploitation remained hidden from view".

Shockingly, it also recounts in the words of the children and young people themselves how "Rather than deal with the perpetrators, the statutory agencies, particularly the police, assigned blame to those who were being abused" (Jay 2022). They were apparently not worthy of protection.

We would also argue that a delivery of public services for vulnerable groups in society through a profit motive is bound to lead to a prioritising of profit for investors as opposed to safety for the vulnerable people the service is meant to protect. The running of children's homes for profit by companies who have been shown to have little regard for the quality of the service offered or the safety and risk aspects of the work (BBC 2022a).

Anne Longfield, the former children's commissioner for England, said the profit-driven care system was failing vulnerable children, with too many accommodated hundreds of miles from their homes and huge amounts of money leaking out of children's services to private shareholders and owners (The Guardian 2022).

So, we can see now taking shape is a landscape of the intersection of racism, poor attitudes towards children, sexist attitudes towards females, institutions failing to take seriously their duty to protect children and young people, and looked after children's services being run for profit. But there may also be another factor here influencing the picture. This requires a consideration of the unconscious factors which inhibit the ability to act with compassion and to apply the law.

We would like to develop some thinking in this chapter about the unconscious factors which may from a psychoanalytic perspective, shed some light on other reasons why children and young people were left unprotected by the agencies which were meant to protect them, despite the known abuse that was taking place. This approach may provide valuable insights.

Scanlon and Adam make the point when discussing the issue of homelessness that "The consequences of society's widespread difficulty with accepting unconscious factors means that individuals are increasingly blamed for their own predicament … There is also ample documented evidence that when they do receive 'health' or 'social care' interventions, these can often appear like 'revenge', 'retaliation' or, at the very least, prejudice and discrimination meted out by practitioners who have become at best unwitting arbiters of 'social worth' and at worst agents of social control acting out society's unconscious hatred of 'them'" (Scanlon and Adam 2019).

It is an exploration of this hatred which can be most productive here, in my opinion, in uncovering the numerous failures of professional services to identify, support, and protect these children and young women from sexual exploitation by men.

Freud, in "Instincts and Their Vicissitudes" (Freud 1915), wrote that "Hate as a relation to objects, is older than love. It derives from the narcissistic ego's primordial repudiation of the external world with its outpouring of stimuli. As an expression of the reaction of unpleasure evoked by objects, it always remains in an intimate relation with the self-preservative instincts… when during the stage of primary narcissism, the object makes its appearance, the second opposite to loving, namely hating, also attains its development. … if the object is a source of unpleasurable feelings, there is an urge which endeavours to increase the distance between the object and the ego and to repeat in relation to the object the original attempt at flight from the external world with its emission of stimuli. We feel the 'repulsion' of the object and hate it; this hate can afterwards be intensified to the point of an aggressive inclination against the object – an intention to destroy it".

Vega Roberts (1994) discusses this in her paper "The Self-imposed Impossible" when she says, "This disregard, even hatred of external reality is typical of the basic assumption mode of group functioning where the task pursued by a group is more meeting of members internal needs than the work task" (p. 112).

Building on this, it is valuable to consider the difficult fact of the deep sense of unease that can be generated in the professional when working with traumatised clients who are challenging and provocative. This is reflected in this passage by Brown (2019): "Maltreated children become 'containers' for a perverse and malign emotional environment through a type of absorptive introjection, taking all that is rotten and corrupt into themselves … taking on the role of 'problem' in a damaging system".

If the reader holds this in mind for a moment and considers some of the comments by Professor Alexis Jay, who gave her views in an interview with the *New York Times* (September 1, 2014):

"When parents reported their daughters missing, it could take 24 hours for the police to turn up, Ms. Jay said. Some parents, if they called in repeatedly, were fined for wasting police time … Some officers and local officials told the investigation that they did not act for fear of being accused of racism. But Ms. Jay said that for years there was an undeniable culture of institutional sexism. Her investigation heard that police referred to victims as 'tarts' and to the girls' abuse as a 'lifestyle choice'… In the minutes of a meeting about a girl who had been raped by five men, a police detective refused to put her into the sexual abuse category, saying he knew she had been '100 percent consensual'. She was 12 … 'These girls were often treated with utter contempt' Ms. Jay said." (Bennhold, 2014)

In her report into the child sexual abuse in Rotherham, South Yorkshire, Professor Jay said that for the first 12 years covered by the inquiry, the "collective failures of political and social leadership were blatant…stark evidence came in 2002, 2003 and 2006 with three reports known to the Police and the Council, which could not have been clearer in their description of the situation in Rotherham. The first of these reports was effectively suppressed" while the other two were "ignored" (Jay 2022).

In my experience in children and adult social care over the last 25 years, we have on occasions come across teams or individuals or case examples in which indifference or hatred has been allowed to ferment within the approach to the children or young people who present with such acute vulnerability and need. Children who are severely neglected or sexually abused can be, as a result of their acute early damage, difficult to work with at times. The work with them can be experienced as unrewarding as they can sometimes see the help they are offered as the problem, as it evokes painful feelings of what has been missing or reminders of their acute vulnerability and precarious existence. Sometimes, they can be highly challenging and provoke powerful feelings in the professional which can be very hard to manage or think about or talk about. In turn, institutions are often designed to dissuade professionals from reflecting on these intractable and messy emotions, so the professional has to face the painful feelings on their own.

This constellation of factors combined with the hatred of the external stimulus to think the unthinkable and disturbing experiences of these children and young people in the context of a societal refusal to grasp the widespread endemic nature of CSE and what Nelson describes as "the most defended of crimes" (Nelson 2016), make a remarkably potent problematic, in which the unthinkable can not only enact itself but evade detection even when it is in plain sight.

Some of the literature in this subject usefully discusses the factors that contribute to the vulnerabilities of these children and young people to sexual exploitation. Some of these factors include family breakdown, previous experiences of abuse, and "concomitant worthlessness and low self-esteem" (Coy 2009), a history of running away and substance misuse. Specific failings in the care system can add to these vulnerabilities such as multiple placement moves within care which are "profoundly destabilising" and undermine their capacity to form trusting relationships. One young woman in this research (Coy 2009) said, "They can show some love or caring, instead of this 'we're moving you there'. They need to stop moving people around like bags of rubbish nobody wants (Christina 21)". For contemporary evidence of this, see the BBC News item from July 2022 about children in care being placed illegally in caravans in BBC (2022b). One can see here the accumulation of factors which can create the conditions under which children and young people, particularly girls and young women, are rendered more vulnerable to CSE. It also illustrates how these failings can contribute to their suffering.

In the face of this depressing picture, thanks to some diligent practice research by key practice researchers in the field, we know what works.

Gladman and Heal (2017) give a thorough description of the components of effective practice in this area (p. 148). There are a number of examples of excellent practices that have arisen around the United Kingdom in response to CSE. Sarah Nelson and Norma Baldwin (Nelson 2016) describe models for practice in community prevention which are evidence based and effective (but despite this they "remain on the margins of mainstream provision within the UK"). Nelson offers the NMCS model (Neighbourhood Mapping for Children's Safety) which "is rooted in the conviction that an overarching view of the needs of communities and neighbourhoods, based on detailed local information and understanding of the links between different sorts of harm to children, is crucial in developing effective child protection strategies" (p. 215).

References

Barnardo's (2014). *Report of the Parliamentary Inquiry into the effectiveness of legislation for tackling child sexual exploitation and trafficking within the UK*. Report-of-the-parliamentary-inquiry-into-the-effectiveness-of-legislation-for-tackling-child-sexual-exploitation-and-trafficking-within-the-uk.pdf

BBC. (2022a). News *"Assaults, Abuse, and Big Profits"*. 9 June 2022. https://www.bbc.co.uk/news/uk-61709572

BBC. (2022b). https://www.bbc.co.uk/news/uk-62127523

Bennhold, K. (2014). *Years of Rape and Utter Contempt in Britain*. The New York Times, Article 1 September 2014. New York.

Brown, G. (2019). *Beyond the Pale*, in Brown, G. Ed *Psychoanalytic Thinking on the Unhoused Mind*. Oxford, Routledge.

Cockbain, E. and Tufail, W. (2020). *Failing Victims, Fuelling Hate: Challenging the Harms of the "Muslim Grooming Gangs" Narrative*. Race & Class. 54(4) (Apr–June 2013). https://doi.org/10.1177/0306396819895727

Coy, M. (2009). *Bags of Rubbish*. Child Abuse Review. 18, 254–266.

Davis, J. (2022). *Adultification bias within child protection and safeguarding* (justiceinspectorates.gov.uk).

Davis, J. (2019). *Where are the black girls in our CSA services, studies and statistics?* Community Care, 19 November 2019. https://www.communitycare.co.uk/2019/11/20/where-are-the-black-girls-in-our-services-studies-and-statistics-on-csa/

Department for Education. (2022). *Working together to safeguard children* – GOV. UK (www.gov.uk).

DoH. (2000). *Report into child prostitution*. child prostitution report (iriss.org.uk).

Drew, J. (2016) *An independent review of South Yorkshire Police's handling of child sexual exploitation 1997–2016*. http://www.drewreview.uk/wp-content/uploads/2016/03/SYP030-Final-report.pdf

Freud, S. (1915). *Instincts and Their Vicissitudes*. Collected Papers, IV. London, Hogarth Press, 1925.

Gladman, A. and Heal, A. (2017). *Child Sexual Exploitation After Rotherham*. London, Jessica Kingsley Publisher.

Goff, P. A., Jackson, M.C., Di Leone, B. A. L., Culotta, C.M., Di Tomasso, N. (2014). *The essence of innocence: Consequences of dehumanizing black children* (apa.org).

Epstein, R, Blake, J.J., and Gonzalez, T. (2017). *Girlhood interrupted: The erasure of black girls' childhood* (georgetown.edu).

Home Office. (2017). *Tackling child sexual exploitation: progress report* – GOV.UK (www.gov.uk).

Jay, A. (2014). *Independent enquiry into child sexual exploitation in Rotherham 1997–2013.* https://www.rotherham.gov.uk/downloads/file/279/independent-inquiry-into-child-sexual-exploitation-in-rotherham#:~:text=Our%20conservative%20estimate%20is%20that,of%20child%20protection%20and%20neglect

Jay, A. (2022). *The independent report into child sexual abuse.* https://www.iicsa.org.uk/index.html#:~:text=The%20Inquiry%20published%20its%20final,survivors%20of%20child%20sexual%20abuse

John (2022). *Child Q – a defining moment for schools* – Institute of Race Relations (irr.org.uk).

Jones, A. and Trottman. J.E. (2009). *Child sexual abuse in the Eastern Caribbean: The report of a study carried out across the eastern Caribbean during the period October 2008 to June 2009* | The British Library (bl.uk).

Letourneau, E.J., Eaton, W.W., Bass, J., Berlin, F.S. and Moore, S.G. (2014). *The Need for a Comprehensive Public Health Approach to Preventing Child Sexual Abuse.* Norwich, Public Health Reports. 129(3), 222–228. University of East Anglia, School of Social Work and Psychosocial Studies.

Mathers, C., Stevens, G. and Mascarenhas, M.G. (2009). *Global health risks: Mortality and burden of disease attributable to selected major risks.* World Health Organization https://www.who.int/publications/i/item/9789241563871

Melrose, M. (2004). *Young People Abused through Prostitution: Some Observations for Practice.* Practice. 16(1), 17–29.

National Child Protection Inspections. (2019). Thematic Report. Available at National Child Protection Inspections: 2019 thematic report – His Majesty's Inspectorate of Constabulary and Fire & Rescue Services (justiceinspectorates. gov.uk).

Nelson, S. (2016). *Tackling Child Sexual Abuse.* Bristol, Policy Press.

NSPCC. (2021). *Statistics on child sexual abuse* | NSPCC Learning (Accessed: September 2023).

Office of National Statistics. (2020). Child Abuse in England and Wales, March 2020 https://www.ons.gov.uk/peoplepopulationandcommunity/crimeandjustice/bulletins/childabuseinenglandandwales/march2020.

PACE. (2019). *Relational Safeguarding Model.* Relational-Safeguarding-Model-2019-digital.pdf (paceuk.info).

Pitts, J. (1997). *'Causes of Youth Prostitution: New Forms of Practice and Political Responses'* in Barrett, D. Ed Child Prostitution in Britain: Dilemmas and Practical Responses. London, The Children's Society.

Roberts. (1994). *The Self-Imposed Impossible Task*, in Obholzer, A. and Roberts V. Eds *The Unconscious at Work.* London, Routledge.

Scanlon, C. and Adam, J. (2019). *Housing Un-Housed Minds*, in Brown, G. Ed *Psychoanalytic Thinking on the Unhoused Mind.* Oxford, Routledge.

Stockholm Declaration. (1996). *The Stockholm Declaration and Agenda for Action.* Available at Microsoft Word – Stockholm A4A.doc (dji.de).

Swann, S. (2000). Helping girls involved in 'prostitution': a Barnardos' experiment. Chapter 14 in Itzin, C. Ed *Home Truths about Child Sexual Abuse: Policy and Practice: A Reader.* London, Routledge.

The Guardian. (2022). *Serious incidents more common in for-profit children's homes in England.* htps://www.theguardian.com/society/2022/jun/28/serious-incidents-more-common-in-for-profit-childrens-homes-in-england

9

SHAME, BLAME AND THE THINKING COMMUNITY

Janine Cherry-Swaine

It defies credulity that large groups of children, more often than not girls, could be subjected to cruelty and contempt, wrapped in a carapace of seduction, groomed, and sexually exploited. Moreover, this can seemingly be hidden in plain sight within communities and services that struggle to come to a realisation of the abuse. As we know, this was the case within such notable towns as Rochdale, Oxford, Telford (Crowther, T 2022), Rotherham (Jay, A 2014), Humberside and many more not specifically named in the public domain. Jay suggested that 1,400 victims could be identified and over 1,000 in Telford going back to the 1980s. Recent reports have suggested that over 16,000 child sexual exploitation victims can be identified in England alone (Edwards, J 2023). This is a disturbing figure which indicates that nationally child sexual exploitation is still very much a problem for services and all of society.

Given the extent of outrage that is triggered by each revelation, and a societal consensus on the need to eradicate it, we need to ask what hinders us in getting to grips with this problem. We need, I think, to regard it as a 'wicked problem' (Grint, K 2005). It is a problem whose complexity creates huge and seemingly insoluble difficulties in the professional and legal networks that attempt to address it. The problem is compounded by the existing difficulties within the individuals, services and communities that it affects.

In this chapter, I will be presenting a series of case examples to illustrate some aspects of this complex problem, and to explain how the consultation service that I run attempts to address it and to mitigate its impact on both staff groups and survivors.

Child sexual exploitation is clearly not constrained to any one area, yet the excruciating extent of the shame that communities are forced to carry when the prevalence has been exposed persuades us to feel that it is contained

DOI: 10.4324/9781003020370-9

and constrained to certain areas. This indicates the power of the unconscious dynamics of splitting and denial that are at play, and the wish to create scape-goats, who can then be vilified: creating the illusion that other areas are free of the problem. For this reason, my case examples will be drawn from communi-ties and staff groups where the prevalence of child sexual exploitation has not been exposed, as well as from various places where it has. To preserve confi-dentiality, these cases are themselves composite examples that explore the im-pact upon individual survivors of their exploitation, of services that support them, and of the professional networks in which these services operate.

A projective system

Child sexual exploitation typically involves a gang mainly consisting of men who get together to recruit young girls to be shared for sexual purposes. The sexual acts often involve extremes of violence, sadism and humiliation. Re-cruitment is achieved through a process of expert grooming, which resembles traditional courtship. Grooming is thus a hidden crime that cannot be easily distinguished, and which can deceive observers as well as the victims and thus go unremarked.

The particular nature of the process of grooming leads to an extraordinarily complex agglomeration of conflicting feelings. Adult survivors have described the initial 'pleasure' and 'enjoyment' at the emotionally attentive and expertly executed courtship, led by attractive young men, seemingly offering themselves to be 'boyfriends' to often vulnerable, lonely young girls. For the children and young women involved, the ensuing 'relationship' is felt at first to be wholly consensual. Although courtship is soon replaced by intimidation, threats and physical abuse, the process typically creates in the victim a confused attach-ment relationship – not unlike that found in many victims of adult domestic abuse. Victims of domestic abuse find it hard to extricate themselves from the projections of a single partner. These are projections that can leave the victims full of shame, blaming themselves and colluding with a process that keeps the abuse secret and isolates them from friends and family.

The victims of child sexual exploitation are recipients of group projections – projections that are exponentially greater than the projections of a single individual – and find it correspondingly harder to extricate themselves from these projections. Their recruitment into the secret, shameful activities of the gang serves similarly to isolate them from their communities. They are faced with a conflict between their previous attachments – which may in themselves be confused and ambivalent – and their attachment to the gang, complicated by feelings of shame and humiliation which are so powerful that they may need to be denied.

As a psychotherapist working with individual survivors, my counter-transference response has informed me of the strength and confusion of these emotions. In my work with staff groups and communities, I am struck by the parallel strength and confusion of emotions engendered in those attempting to work with them, which can affect me as strongly as my work with individual survivors. This is a measure of the power of the projective system created by the process. As a psychoanalytic thinker, I assume that gangs of sexual abusers come together because of their own unconscious need to rid themselves of powerful negative emotions. They project into their victims, a toxic mix that they themselves have been unable to process. Evidence to support this view. It is widely reported, for instance, that some of the convicted abusers came from an Asian heritage. They often come from generations of traumatised adults previously displaced from historical conflict zones and subsequently marginalised and humiliated by their adopted country. Perhaps they and their families have themselves felt seduced and tricked by false promises of security and prosperity that have not been fulfilled by the reality of their experiences of Western capitalism.

However, there has been very little research about the perpetrators of this form of abuse other than that which is written in newspapers or in court proceedings. The impression is that the criminals are either full of guile, brazen or deny knowledge: smiling young men who admonish social workers, accusing them of failing to protect young girls only later to be charged with the crime themselves. Or the opposite; mug shots of older men from criminal proceedings that give nothing away about who they were in their younger days when the abuse took place. While it is not within the scope of this chapter to explore the predicament of the abusers, it is likely that a fuller understanding of their histories would greatly aid our work in preventing continuing abuse and untangling its impact. We already know that a greater knowledge of the histories of both partners helps us to better understand and prevent domestic abuse.

The projective parcel

In the absence of fuller research, I would suggest that the nature of child sexual exploitation provides copious evidence of what is being projected. Child sexual exploitation involves the projection of shame, which must then be denied and kept secret. Through the process of grooming, victims are typically tricked into becoming complicit with sadistic sexual acts. They are corrupted and humiliated and sometimes forced into recruiting new victims. This process leaves survivors with an agglomeration of conflictual feelings which they find almost impossible to untangle. A messy parcel of feelings that has been passed to them and that they find themselves passing on in turn. The less able they are to make sense of their tangled feelings, the more likely they are to deny them and project the whole agglomerated parcel into others.

The abuse often occurs within a close community. People know one another, but those around them don't know that it is happening. The victims are made to feel like aliens within their own peer groups. Abusers and victims are often drawn together through an unconscious recognition of an experience of alienation that they have in common. Abusers are drawn to victims vulnerable to being shamed and humiliated. Victims often have a similarly denied experience of projected toxicity as a result of childhood abuse, abandonment, disability or sometimes simply an ordinary mischance that has set them apart from their peer group.

Because these accreted experiences of toxic projections have not been digested and processed either by the abusers or by the victims, the projections into the community and into its services have an aggregated force that is particularly hard for staff groups to think about or to contain. Like the abusers and the victims, staff groups and communities find themselves humiliated and powerless, the target of outrage and blame. This is evidenced by the response of the press and the flurry of resignations that follow new exposures.

In what follows, I will attempt to describe through case material something of how this plays out for the staff groups that work with individual survivors and attempt to cope with the complexity of their projections.

Working with staff groups

The services I have worked with include a variety of National Health Service Social Care, Housing, and Voluntary Sector organisations in various towns. When I started working, I was astonished – given the widespread nature of the media coverage in some of these areas – to find that it was almost impossible to locate many adult survivors of child sexual exploitation – as if they remained a 'shameful secret' (Crowther, T 2022). It took time and patience to unearth names and details. I soon discovered that in order to do so I had to be hyper-sensitive to the issues of blame, shame and scapegoating, feared and sometimes experienced by workers in relation to the individual victims.

I also noticed an initial misguided wish to find a way of treating the impact of child sexual exploitation as if it was a distinct layer that could be eradicated and split off from any pre-existing trauma and complexity. Any need to address the previous history of victims that might have made them more vulnerable to exploitation was denied. This led to fragmented thinking and non-collaborative service responses. I quickly came to the conclusion that this was a reaction to the nature and complexity of the problem that services were attempting to deal with.

My decision to work consultatively was based on my understanding that the projection of blame, shame, and scapegoating needed to be countered by a group response. Professional networks needed to collaborate to process. Professionals collectively needed to understand and detoxify the complex parcel of emotions that had been projected into individual survivors and through them into the staff groups attempting to help them. The team of consultative clinicians that I have gathered together and trained to work with the professional networks has been hugely successful in supporting survivors through supporting their workers.

The following vignette offers an example of what can be projected into staff groups and individual staff members by the nature of what individual survivors are carrying – and of how these staff groups and staff members can be supported in their painful and difficult work.

Jane

A project worker, whom I will call Jane, asked for help from a multi-agency group of workers. Very quickly and shockingly for the group, she began sharing graphic and sadistic details of the story of a victim being sexually abused by a series of men. The details were very explicit and involved a re-telling of the exact narrative that had been shared with her by the victim. The group members later reported feeling frozen when they heard this. They felt shocked and in a bind. On the one hand, they did not want to turn away or prevent Jane from continuing with her narrative, as they were concerned that this would seem unprofessional. On the other hand, they were filled with a mixture of really unbearable emotions when they listened to her: perverse sexual excitement, shame and rage. We can see here an echo of the victim's feelings. She wanted to appear 'cool' and unfazed by her 'boyfriend's' demands. Like the group members, she was also shocked, humiliated and perversely excited.

The group members responded by turning their anger and outrage on to Jane; they felt that she had abused the group by exposing them to pornographic content, 'awful stuff' as they called it, that they had unwittingly been forced to consume. Jane was shamed and ashamed, blamed for being sexually provocative rather than understood as having been overwhelmed by her client's projections. The group's response to Jane's presentation – the 'awful stuff' – threatened to disturb a culture of cooperation and partnership that had just begun to be established in this multi-agency forum. However, with consultative help, both Jane and the group were able to see and work through what had happened to them. The group's incoherent rage at feeling the shame of being made to be complicit in their exposure to sexually explicit material and their attempt to blame and scapegoat Jane were transformed into a very powerful emotional learning experience. Supported, they could come together to express and articulate traumatic content appropriately, filtering out the sadism and the perverse sexual projections without denying their existence.

Without consultation, the original trauma of sexual exploitation risked being catapulted through the system, fracturing emotional boundaries and psychological defences and leading to the scapegoating of one member – Jane – and a refusal to take on board and to address the 'awful stuff', the content that she was trying to communicate to them.

Responses

If staff groups and professionals can stay with the 'awful stuff', a number of responses can be identified, and patterns can begin to emerge – a developing framework that makes it easier to think in the face of the extreme feelings engendered by the trauma of child sexual exploitation. The learning and experience that I and my team have gained from consultation to staff groups can be described through a series of case examples.

The emotional legacy for individual survivors of child sexual exploitation is complex, and survivors cope in a variety of ways as they begin to process the experience. The descriptions here are, of course, over-simplified but serve to illustrate the stages that victims may go through in coming to terms with what has happened to them – the 'awful stuff' that nobody wants to think about. At first, the predominant feelings of shock, outrage, fury and shame are likely to be denied, and the individual may insist on maintaining an attachment to the grooming gang and may reject offers of help. This was the case with Tilly.

Tilly

Tilly was fourteen when she eventually entered a children's home. She had been known to social services for some years as a result of parental neglect. She was subsequently found to have been passed around by groups of men, returning to them time and time again despite the degradation and abuse that she suffered at their hands.

On her first day of arrival in a small, detached house on a quiet residential street, she immediately opened the windows and screamed a stream of obscenities in the direction of the elderly neighbour: she then invited him into the house to have sex with her and the staff.

The staff were mortified. They were extremely embarrassed by her and dreaded the thought of being seen in public with her. The owners felt threatened as any complaints would affect their rating with Ofsted.

In consultation sessions, the staff described her as 'excited', 'deceitful' and 'animalistic' some of the time. At other times, she exhibited moments of unfocussed passivity, as if disconnected from reality and caught up in her own internal world. They admitted that she was hard to warm to. The situation worsened when they had reason to suspect that she had been 'tampering' with the shared food in the fridge. They were really worried that she had poisoned the food and that they might be harmed. Such was the level of anxiety that they insisted to her social worker that she needed to refer Tilly to a secure unit. They did not feel able to continue her placement in the home.

In the consultation sessions, we became more able to discuss and understand the 'awful stuff', the specific abuse that she had suffered, and how she was filled with the degradation emanating from the abusers. Their anxiety decreased. They withdrew their insistence that Tilly be placed in a secure unit and agreed that she could stay. They began to realise that Tilly felt that her mind and body had been poisoned by her experiences. She had a sparseness of pre-existing stability and love to draw upon prior to the abuse to counteract the poison and tether her to reality. Through a period of consultation, the staff were able to see that they too felt that they had been poisoned: filled up with a host of uncomfortable feelings, 'awful stuff' being projected into them by Tilly. This had led them to believe that Tilly was poisoning their food. As they worked through a process of articulating these feelings, sorting them, and making sense of them, the staff group was able to begin to decipher what had been projected into them. This was a process of emotional decontamination that Tilly was not yet able to manage on her own behalf. However, it made the difference between staying in the home and going to a secure unit.

Gradually, over about a year, Tilly became more settled into a routine and started to attend college. She became more organised in her thinking and in her relationships. The risky behaviour decreased, and she seemed to be less in thrall to her abusers. She was able to accept the support of her staff group rather than identify with the abusers. She began showing this in her own ability to contain and manage her own feelings rather than project them into others. When a new child was introduced to the home, Tilly could admit how she felt troubled at having to share her staff – an example of her growing ability to be more realistically in touch with the normal conflicts of ordinary life.

Tilly is an example of a victim who retreated into dissociative states, denying her own emotional reality and projecting her unbearable feelings into the staff. Because her identification with her abusers was understood and processed by the staff around her, she was able to make contact with her own emotional reality and grow authentic relationships with those around her.

For adult survivors, the oscillation between identification with the abusers and an attempt to reach out for help may become entrenched and it can be harder for professionals to intervene. They seem to embody both the abuser and the victim, and they can become both the accused and the accusers.

Helen

Helen was in her late thirties. She had been introduced to drugs at thirteen as a result of sexual exploitation. She continued to use drugs to block out her nightmares. The professional network around her had found her difficult at first – it had seemed hard to make a properly empathic relationship with her. They had eventually warmed to her and worked hard to make progress. They were devastated when it was revealed that, having been groomed herself, she was suspected of having later procured other young girls for the gang and subsequently charged by the police. They felt blindsided by this news and could not find a way of joining these two versions of Helen.

In the course of consultation, they admitted feeling betrayed by her, even duped, doubting the warmth and attachment that had developed and struggling to disentangle the complexities of their own responses. They discussed the nature of grooming and the complexities of the conflictual feelings that had been projected into Helen. They thought about the topsy-turvy world of the victim and of how a victim might try to escape from being the one at the bottom by any means if it kept them alive and rescued them from sadistic attack, powerlessness and painful humiliation. They were able to empathise with the heartbreak of Helen's story while fully recognising that she had lured others in to take her place and undergo the same sadistic treatment.

Helen had lived with the impact of child sexual exploitation for some years and had not had sufficient help to process her conflictual feelings. Instead, she seemed to have split her identity: one part of her appeared to be authentic in her presentation as an innocent victim to the professional network. Another hidden part of her retained a firm identification with the abusive gang. For many victims, the experience of sexual exploitation becomes embodied through an entrenched identification with the abusers that is hard for them to acknowledge.

Gail

Gail, in my next example, was younger than Helen. She oscillated between her attempts to reach out for help and her attempts to avoid any kind of rescue. But in her case, the conflict was more overt, and because her early history was better known, it was easier for the professionals to make sense of her behaviour.

Gail was in her mid-twenties and had lived in around eight different places in a similar number of months. She was constantly being given notice, absconding, or getting involved in some disaster that warranted a move. She would make what seemed to be good starts – warm relationships with housing support staff, for instance – and then she would flee and lose these relationships. She was also in and out of domestic abuse relationships and financially vulnerable. This volatility was affecting every aspect of her health and welfare: it meant that she was inaccessible to her GP[1] who was unable to offer her any onward referrals for checkups.

This transitory existence was matched by her mood, which was up and down like a 'rollercoaster'. When it was disclosed that the man who had been put in prison for grooming and exploiting her was soon to be released, the anxiety amongst the professionals heightened. Her workers began advocating strongly for her to have a mental health service to help with her depressive and self-harm risks. The staff became angry with faceless mental health services and social care for refusing to provide Gail with a 'better' service and 'better' placements, and assumed that she, and they, would be abandoned.

Initially, staff were frustrated and angry, if not insulted, at being offered consultation to understand their concerns about Gail in context. There were reservations about calling a wider network meeting with both past and present housing support staff, but eventually, they agreed to a series of consultative meetings between them and the wider professional network. During these meetings, a fuller chronology of Gail's history was re-visited, which helped her current workers to better understand how transience had been a feature throughout Gail's life, right from being an infant to being a child in multiple families. The details of her early childhood were very painful for all to hear but enabled them to understand that Gail did not expect to stay anywhere for long. In a way, she perpetuated a series of new starts where the 'grass always promised to be greener'. They also realised that in some subtle but powerful ways, organisations had historically been unconsciously playing into this.

In the end, the group met for more than a year. There were consistent members with some people joining for a particular reason, but in each meeting, the participants would share observations in turn and consider in detail the presenting issue in Gail's life. Group members would share in confidence their own emotional responses, and how they felt towards Gail. Sometimes, they were acutely ambivalent, and they admitted that they hated her for going back to men who harmed her. The consultants were sensitive in their handling of these painful counter-transference responses. This helped the staff to admit that, on occasion, they had a strong desire to be rid of her, as she caused them to feel so much pain, guilt, and inadequacy because of their inability to protect her.

In a sense, the group was undergoing psychotherapy on Gail's behalf. The group had learned to manage the consistency that hitherto Gail had not been able to manage herself. In particular, they resisted fleeing from the problems by onward referrals to 'better' placements or 'better' services. After some time, the group looked back and was astonished to notice the changes that had taken place: Gail had not moved once during this period, and her health and well-being had significantly improved. The staff were proud of their work with her. The network around Gail had been able to help her both physically and emotionally.

It was significant that Gail's problems included unexplained illnesses, which were a source of concern to her GP. For many victims, the experience of child sexual exploitation becomes embodied not only through an entrenched identification with the abusers but also through the physical sequelae of unprocessed emotional pain. Self-harm, suicide and physical illnesses are common amongst survivors. Susan, for instance, withdrew from the world and seemed just to give up. She disengaged from all offers of professional help.

She eventually died of a failure of her internal organs for which the hospital where she was taken could offer no explanation.

The legal system

I hope that through these case examples, I have illustrated one element in particular, the shame and conflictual feelings of the survivors. There are many problems that are the consequence of child sexual exploitation. Through a systematised grooming process somewhat akin to brainwashing, victims have been tricked into colluding in their own abuse. They have been complicit, and they struggle to free themselves of their identification with their abusers. It can be hard for them to maintain their innocence to themselves, let alone to a court. Seeking and gaining justice is a complicated matter, and separating guilt from innocence may not be easy, as Helen's case illustrates. However, for just this reason, a court process, and a verdict delivered by the Criminal Justice System affirming the guilt of their abusers, is of huge psychological importance for victims. It exonerates them, providing public vindication and restoring them to full membership of their communities.

Achieving justice in cases of rape, or multiple rapes, such as many of the victims have suffered, may also be impossible for other reasons. Many women who have attempted to stick with the long investigations that have been a feature of life in several of the towns affected have ultimately been told that there will be 'No Further Action'. Prosecution Services have had to conclude that a case cannot be pursued in the theatre of the court. Sometimes, the necessary evidence is not available or not sufficient. Women are often unable to describe the rapists. They couldn't bear to look them in the face. Sometimes, the emotional vulnerability of the witness may indicate that it is unlikely that a trial will reach the desired conclusion or that the witness will emerge safely from the ordeal.

Police officers and investigative teams in this situation can find themselves feeling full of guilt. They feel that they and the system have failed the witnesses, giving them hope but then letting them down and seeming to abandon them. This dynamic can be all the more powerful because of the painful emotional work involved for the victim in presenting her case. I'll give one example.

Lesley

Lesley had just about survived into her thirties with a history of repeated overdoses and frequent visits to Accident and Emergency. She was the mother of two children, who had been in and out of the care of the local authority; much as she had herself as a child.

In a consultation to the professional network, the criminal justice representative, John, explained the current circumstances. Lesley's' evidence was being scrutinised to see what inconsistencies it contained and whether it was sufficiently robust to allow Lesley to be considered a 'reliable witness'. The group doubted her capacity to withstand harsh cross-examination, especially given the level and frequency of the dissociative states from which she suffered and her unconvincing and chaotic presentation. This was hugely disappointing for all the professionals, and especially for Lesley's support worker, Nancy. The group became very depressed. Nancy reported that Lesley, despite her vulnerable health and the risks involved, was adamant that she should give her evidence in court and have the abuse fully acknowledged. In the subsequent discussion, she and John were able to share some very detailed observations of Lesley. They observed that she came across as disconcertingly childlike, giggling and seeming much smaller than her real height. They admitted to feeling very protective of her, as though she were a very little girl. The group wondered whether they were being unconsciously pulled into acting towards her as if they were parents of a very small and sexually innocent child.

Members of the group wondered whether their recognition and acceptance of Lesley's childlike dependency had supported Lesley in overcoming her conflictual identification with the abusers but whether it was now hindering her in achieving the more adult autonomy she needed if she was to give evidence in court. Nancy and John acknowledged that they had somehow become confused about the reality of her chronological age. She did, after all, manage some degree of maturity in her wish to be a better parent for her children. They wondered how they could use this insight to support and encourage the more mature part of Lesley's personality. How could they help her to communicate more authoritatively as the adult she was rather than to retreat into a state of infantile mindlessness? The group understood that this could only be achieved if the workers themselves were able to recognise and stay alongside the sexually mature adolescent Lesley that had been drawn into collusion with the abuse while still recognising and sympathising with the little girl Lesley who had longed to be loved and wanted at any price. Through this work, Lesley's professional network was eventually able to support her in achieving a guilty verdict.

It requires a sophisticated relational effort on the part of the professional support services and the community around them to find a way to consistently assert and communicate their innocence to survivors of exploitation. They need to confirm that their stories are believed and that, despite their collusion, they are not to blame. However, although it can be very helpful to victims to have 'had their day in court', this is not always achievable. Where it is not, such a professional network can provide alternative vindication. Because this is in the context of longer lasting and ongoing relationships, it may contribute to a more substantial outcome and an alternative and more healing legacy.

A system wide model

The examples I have given, and the model of consultation I and my team provide, are not unfamiliar to child psychotherapists, organisational therapists and consultants working to support teams and services. What may be less common is the opportunity to provide coverage across the wider landscape of services that support victims.

Sexual abuse of any kind, but particularly child sexual exploitation, involves a very closed system in order to exist. A consultation and training offer ensures that the staff who support victims are part of an open system of collaborative learning; this stands in contrast to the dynamics of abuse. Where the whole of a community over a wide geographical area has been shamed and publicly humiliated, an approach that serves to detoxify this shame and understands the origins of the projections has many advantages. The model my team uses has grown incrementally, supported not only by the perseverance of commissioners to seek funding for this project but also by their willingness to share their honest concerns about their communities. It has been based upon a great deal of trust earned over several years by the avoidance of any hint of shaming or of 'pointing the finger'.

The crucial importance of this was brought home to me once when, after a group that I had facilitated, the senior manager said, 'that went really well'. Pleased with this comment I asked her what she thought had been most helpful. 'You didn't tell anyone off!', she said. I was a little disappointed as this seemed a low bar for the success of my work, but it did give me an indication of how powerful the expectations were of being blamed and shamed. Cooper (2015) talks about the 'persecutory anxiety' arising out of the 'fear of public humiliation' where there is organisational failure. It takes a great deal of time and emotional effort for organisations to work through these projections.

In the case of towns blighted by child sexual exploitation, a whole geographical area containing many services is affected. This impacts not only their relationship with themselves but also their relationships with other services and with how they collaborate and link up together. The potential for splitting between services and for projecting all the problems, the shame and the blame into one scapegoated location is high. People who suffer from complex presentations, with or without sexual exploitation as a factor, depend upon services working well together and being compassionate towards one another. Therefore, the advantages of working to support the whole of the workforce covering the geographical spread encourage reciprocity. It mitigates against the sense of being passed on or being dropped, be it survivor or professional. It helps people to sustain their hope and their energies in the face of the emotional chaos and fragmentation that is caused by the shame of their sexual exploitation.

Developing a networked model of consultation means that schools which have perpetrators' children and survivors' children in the same playgrounds and classrooms, and where their families meet at the school gates, are able to seek support to think about seemingly intractable issues. They can find help to work with children and families who have been affected by generational trauma whether the context is as a result of their father being charged and shunned by his community or their mother struggling to manage court appearances.

The spread of consultation across services whether they be voluntary or statutory, criminal justice, housing, drug and alcohol, mental health, social work or schools or a combination of services, has enabled the problem to be located in the abuse and not the work. Shame is understood in context rather than projected. The Telford report mentions the offer of individual counselling for staff employed within services that have failed. This is a noble attempt to notice the impact of taking away the secrecy while acknowledging the risk of exposure. However, there is an advantage in having a work-based system of consultation to staff groups to explore their work and the impact of it. The consultation locates the problem in the emotionally difficult work and its concomitant projections rather than suggesting that it is located in the psychopathology of the individual.

As you will surmise, working across a geographical area with many staff groups requires a team of professionals working cohesively together to provide congruent interventions. While the work is underpinned by a systems psychodynamic approach, the individual team members are drawn from a variety of professional backgrounds. This brings a richness of differing viewpoints as well as reflects the multi-professional nature of the work around victims. Internal staff consultation and team support are vital when there is a risk of vicarious trauma. The team does not work directly with the victims, but I hope I have illustrated here the infectiousness of the toxicity of trauma. It passes so easily from one group to another and risks replicating the very dynamics that we are working to mitigate (Cardona, F 2020) (Moylan, D 2019). Our team has needed to engage in a committed exploration of its own counter-transference responses in order to help other staff groups to do the same.

Conclusion

Casey (2015) doubted mental health services' capacity to respond to the distress and the trauma experienced by victims of child sexual exploitation and their families. She was correct: a traditional approach to mental health support alone is likely to be frustrated in those places affected. In my view, the challenge posed by the fact that victims are spread across various services, rather than presenting a hindrance to supporting them, can, in fact, provide an opportunity to establish a networked approach. Survivors with an enduring emotional complexity can then be provided with a more efficient and responsive offer, bespoke to their needs. The staff who support them can be nurtured rather than risk being shamed in their turn.

Consultation of the kind I have described applies 'a methodology for using counter-transference to help an organisation as a whole, just as (psychotherapists have) been taught to use it to help an individual' (Sprince, J 2002). This methodology has the great merit of helping staff to understand that their uncomfortable feelings of shame, humiliation, confusion, rage and impotence are not solely their own. They form part of a projective parcel, which if left unpacked and unprocessed threatens the cohesion and well-being of individuals, services and communities alike. Instead of concealing such feelings, professionals can learn to explore them in order to make sense of the complex problems that they and their communities are struggling with. They can detoxify this parcel and help others to do so too.

It is my assertion that working across the system consultatively is the therapeutic intervention of choice to support those traumatised individuals who present the most complex problems. They have the greatest difficulty accessing services and present a public health challenge to workers and to the community as a whole. Staff consultation contributes to an emotional experience becoming more coherent, and a foundation for emotional health (Fonagy, P 2003). It works to reverse the tendency towards fragmentation and contributes towards confidence, resilience and self-compassion both in staff groups and in those whom they support.

Acknowledgements

I would like to recognise the help of survivors of child sexual exploitation in giving direction to this work and the commitment and trust of colleagues, including commissioners, from across the various networks. Also, for the steadfast support of Jenny Sprince who has helped me process and attend to 'the awful stuff' in various places over the years, I would like to say thank you.

Note

1 GP is a commonly used UK abbreviation for General Practitioner

References

Cardona, F (2020) The team as a sponge: How the nature of the task affects the behaviour and mental life of a team, in Work Matters: Consulting to Leaders and Organisations in the Tavistock Tradition. Oxon: Routledge.
Casey, L (2015) *Report of the inspection Rotherham Metropolitan Borough Council:* Ministry of Housing, Communities and Local Government. London.

Cooper, A (2015) 'Containing Tensions: Psychoanalysis and modern policy making'. Juncture Vol 22 (No 2) 157–163 Wiley online. https://doi.org/10.1111/j.2050-5876.2015.00852.x

Crowther, T., Chair. (2022) Report of the Independent Inquiry Telford Childhood Sexual Exploitation. Commissioned by: London, Eversheds Sutherland (Intl.) LLP

Edwards, J (2023) Child Exploitation: A Hidden crisis. Barnardo's Briefing paper.

Fonagy, P (2003) 'The development of borderline personality disorder in early attachment relationships: A theory and some evidence'. Psychoanalytic Enquiry Vol 23 (No 3) 412–459.

Grint K (2005) 'Problems, problems, problems: The social construction of leadership'. Human Relations Vol 58 No 11 1467–1494.

Jay, A (2014) Independent Inquiry into Child Sexual Exploitation in Rotherham 1997–2013. Rotherham Metropolitan Borough Council

Moylan, D (2019) The dangers of contagion, in A Obholzer, V Roberts (eds) The Unconscious at Work: A Tavistock Approach to Making Sense of Organisational Life. London: Routledge.

Sprince, J (2002) 'Developing containment: Psychoanalytic consultancy to a therapeutic community for traumatised children'. Journal of Child Psychotherapy Vol 28 No 2 147–161 Oxon: Routledge.

10

ABUSE AND EXPLOITATION IN GROUPS AND ORGANISATIONS

A psychoanalytic psychiatrist's perspective

Judith Trowell

There has been growing awareness for a long time that abuse and exploitation in groups and organisations is a serious problem. It was under cover, and it emerged with high-profile cases where there has been an emphasis on the race of the perpetrators. However, it has been occurring in society over many years in a range of settings – for example see the Cleveland Inquiry Report, Butler-Sloss (1988). Interestingly, it has been ignored, or those in responsible positions have chosen to turn a blind eye.

One might wonder why it has been so hard to recognise. It could be that if a carer has been abused as a child, they cannot allow themselves to see what is happening to children in their care. Perhaps if they do then they have to recall what happened to them as children and it is too painful to contemplate. The dynamics of this process is worth consideration because it reflects on those in senior positions in health, social care, police, and education. For example, in Rotherham, the voluntary sector had to raise concerns that statutory organisations were unable, over many years, to confront.

There are also those more privileged young people, for example, boys who are in church choirs or boarding schools often within a religious foundation. Sexual Abuse and sexual exploitation occur anywhere and are opportunistic. The main abuser is driven by his own sexual addiction and determination to overcome obstacles. In all cases, the perpetrators use pressure to ensure their secret is sustained. The victims are encouraged to feel special. The bribes are increased, and threats may be unspoken, or when verbalised, the implication is that no one will believe their word against an upright member of society. The perpetrators themselves have a range of positions. Most have marriages. Some have church positions. Some are paedophiles with strong sexual impulses particularly for pubertal

DOI: 10.4324/9781003020370-10

young people. Others are flattered to be included in the group and enjoy the sexual availability. This type of sexual activity is a form of addictive behaviour, and this is so for perpetrators and victims. It is a flight from unhappiness into excitement.

Some clinical examples

A specialist NHS[1] clinic dealing with complex abuse cases discovered that, in a large suburban church, a choir master had been abusing the young choristers. He had been sacked and the families were outraged. These were predominantly middle-class boys, mainly white, whose families were very involved and supportive of the church. The boys described how they were made to feel special, asked to help with small tasks, and invited into the choirmaster's room. Often, they were given treats after choir practice: biscuits and sweets. The boys were between 10 and 12 years old.

The choirmaster gained his sexual satisfaction by using the boys in practical tasks. A number of boys were very distressed and had self-doubt. They believed they had brought it on themselves, so alongside the shame was the horror that people would know and what might happen to them in the future. They were not obviously vulnerable but felt damaged and needed help as did the families. One boy became very depressed and muttered about life not being worth living. He needed intensive treatment to aid his recovery.

Abuse may be uncovered when a child is referred to child mental health services – perhaps for other reasons. This may puncture the glamour, and children may become disturbed or distressed.

In a large city local authority where I did some consultation, there were many children in care of the local authority. There were also a fair number of families with lone mothers and, somewhere, children were out roaming the streets. These young people, mainly girls, linked up with men, many from Eastern European countries, who had settled in the area. The girls were befriended by these men, given a good time in flash cars and apparent money to spend. The men were also into alcohol and drugs, cocaine, heroin, and amphetamines. Soon the girls were involved too and dependent on the drugs. A man would spend time with a girl and insist he loved her. Often, the girl moved in with him. Slowly, he would encourage her to have sex with his 'friends'. When she objected, he would suggest it proved how much she loved him. Later, if she declined, he could become violent.

These men were abusing the girls, but the major issue was exploitation, using the girls to run their prostitution business. They were pimping the girls. Often, the girl still believed the man loved her. It was painful and desperate to see these young women who had no one to care for them or protect them. Social workers had given up. If there was a mother or family member around, they felt overwhelmed and powerless.

I ran an NHS clinic study offering treatment to sexually abused girls. Of this group of girls, most had been abused by family members, friends, or neighbours. However, a small number were more seriously damaged, were in care and were having difficulties in all areas of their lives. The details of their backgrounds revealed they had been living in households where there were drugs and alcohol. Mothers were involved in prostitution. These girls, between 8 and 12 years old, had become involved in sexual activity in the household, used by their mothers' clients.

The girls were struggling, mostly labelled as slow learners, and unable to function at school. Their behaviour was impulsive, violent at times, and they ran away. At other times, they were very frightened, had panic attacks, and harmed themselves. The study offered treatment, and these girls received once weekly psychoanalytic psychotherapy or group therapy for a year. There was an improvement overall, but this subgroup subsequently needed intensive therapy or specialist residential therapeutic placement.

I was involved with two other larger scale referrals. A large number of boys and young men were referred who had attended a special physical activities school in the country. The boys had been in trouble with frequent minor offences. The hope had been that they could respond to the different atmosphere and life at the school. By the time of referral, some were in prison, but the majority were offered an appointment. A story emerged of a headmaster and a deputy head who were at the head of a pyramid. Older boys who had been sexually abused on arrival at the school were the procurers for the head and deputy and were able to abuse the younger boys themselves. These older boys and young men were either broken and suicidal (there had been suicides) or in prison following violent offences. One remarked. 'We will all end up in prison or dead'. Some came and told their story and left. They had been sent to the school to help them. Their rage, humiliation, and feeling of betrayal were overwhelming. They were offered treats, cigarettes, town leave, and alcohol, initially for sex, later for bringing younger boys to them. They were scornful and contemptuous of the younger boys (it was some of the younger boys who had raised the alarm). For a few, some sadness emerged for themselves and the others. Most of these young men and boys disappeared. A few were helped by their local authorities.

It was distressing to see the younger boys. Some attended short term. A few managed to engage for longer-term work. These boys often had returned to families that were mobilised and could help them. They felt betrayed, anxious, fearful, and hopeless, but they had been sexually aroused and sought out sex. The underlying problems that led to the school placement also remained. The individuals and families needed help, but also, as a group, they had a strong sense of the need for justice. They blamed the head and deputy. The older boys and men felt they were as much to blame as the staff.

The second such referral involved a number of young women who were causing concern and who were assessed as seriously abused. They were also addicted to drugs and alcohol and had expensive gadgets, clothes, and jewellery. Some of them were suicidal. These cases were investigated. The professionals involved became very worried but then the professionals were attacked and denigrated by leading community members. It was possible eventually to uncover a group activity organised by a prominent member of the local society. A group of men used remote buildings for group sex, the girls were picked up and driven to the location. Younger men were encouraged to join the group with offers of promotion at work but then found it hard to leave. The girls were given a range of treats. When they presented, these girls were overwhelmed by shame, despair, and hopelessness but, on the surface, were impulsive, defiant, and full of bravado.

Some needed inpatient admission; others returned to school, others could not. The professionals who had been involved were finally acknowledged but many took early retirement. They were left depressed and defeated that it took so long for them to be seen as supporting and protecting these girls. They were burnt out, exhausted, relieved it was being dealt with but felt they had had enough. If they worked again it needed to be somewhere less stressful. In all these cases, what was needed was a multidisciplinary team involving child and adolescent mental health, social services, school, and the police to handle the intense emotions, deal with the threats and sustain the focus on discovering what was going on for the children.

The impact on individuals

A well-presented man of about 45 years consulted me and came once weekly. He was married with 2 children, 17 years and 13 years old, and he was in a senior position at work doing fairly well and comfortable financially. The main problem was his difficulties with his wife. He was very close to his two sons and loved doing outdoor activities with them, walking, climbing, and mountaineering. He wanted to go sailing and to buy a small boat. The three of them also went skiing. None of these activities involved his wife. She was complaining, either asking if she could come too, or could they do different things which they could do all together. This had led to problems in their relationship. He did not really want physical intimacy and she was upset about this too. He talked about how unreasonable he found her.

I had to ask several times about his childhood. He was reluctant to say much. His parents had been comfortable and he had been brought up by a nanny, although he spent a lot of time with his parents. They did things as a family – he had a younger brother. At seven years, he went to a boarding prep school which was ok. He had liked it there.

Later, he went to a large public boarding school. He was unhappy there and repeatedly asked his parents if he could leave. The staff said he was doing fine academically, and his parents encouraged him to stay. I wondered with him what was problematic, what was he finding distressing. More than six months later, he came in, gritted his teeth, and said I had stirred everything up and he needed to talk. He remained standing as he talked about the sexual activity he had been involved in at school. Initially as a younger boy, his house master had invited my patient to his room, masturbating mutually, and then anal penetration by the house master. Later, in the sixth form, a number of boys and the master had been sexually active all with each other, penetrating and being penetrated. He said by the end he enjoyed it, liked it, and wanted it, although initially, he had wanted to get away.

He did not sit down as he had usually done. He thought I might object to such a disgusting person sitting on my chair. He felt dirty, ashamed, and quite shocked at what he had remembered, particularly that he had enjoyed quite a lot of it. Nevertheless, he repeated he had been desperate to leave the school. Further work continued for about eighteen months as he tried to make sense of it and his current situation. He felt quite strongly he was homosexual and visited some gay bars. Finally, he talked to his wife and they considered divorce, but they saw a couples therapist and were able to work through the issues as best they could. They were friends and could support each other and parent their sons. It remained unclear how they might meet their needs and what the future might hold.

A second individual, a young man of just 19 years came to see me. He was part of a school referral. He had been at the school for four years and had left two years ago. He had remained connected to the school and some of the other boys and young men. He looked shabby and dishevelled. He was desperate. His eyes had dark rings around. He was a pasty colour with sores on his face from cuts whilst shaving. His hair was spiky and needed a wash. His clothes were not bad but did not fit him. He insisted he was not on drugs, just struggling, but he did have a drink in the evening. He was living in a hostel and did not have any contact with his birth family. He said the other boys and men were his family. He lived on benefits and smoked about 40 cigarettes a day. He said he had an idea of doing gardening, out in the open air, but he could not get up and attend regularly and so had lost his place on a training scheme. He tried to dull his memories of his time at the school with drink and cigarettes, and then said if it was bad, he used hash. He was reluctant to talk about what had happened – he felt his life had been ruined and he was finished. He said he felt guilty about how he had used the younger boys and encouraged them to join in. He used to feel triumphant, high, excited, and he loved going out to the local town to buy cigarettes and other treats. He felt terrible now. He was never going to have a life. He had been sent there because he needed help, and this had made him worse. He felt hopeless. Many of the others were in prison, some had killed themselves. All were violent to themselves or others. He was very angry but what was the point; it could not be undone now. He came for five appointments and links were made with voluntary organisations including Alcoholics Anonymous. Survivors UK for sexually abused men gave him a mentor to support him. Sadly, he then disappeared and could not be found by any agency. We all tried. He had continued to be angry and hopeless although he did indicate telling his story helped a little, but nothing could take it away. Then he vanished completely.

Reflections

Thinking about these examples, how can we understand them? What is striking is how hard it is to be aware, to see what may be happening in front of one. Given the last institutional example, if you do suspect and start to explore, it is easy for the professionals to become vilified. The implication is that they have a problem, a dirty mind, or much worse. The sexual drive is known to be very powerful, life and death. Both examples involve sexuality in every aspect even when it is not apparent. There is an element of sexual interest and curiosity in all aspects of life.

But sexuality is combined with power, assertiveness, or aggression. This is needed in normal sexual relationships but easily becomes corrupted and can lead to sadism or masochism. Sex does involve love, but the element of sadism or masochism can become ends in themselves. The corrupted urge leads to lies, deviousness, ruthlessness, and disregard for the other. This other becomes an object because most forms of sexuality involve another. Even masturbation involves another in the mind. Where there is abuse, the sexual need overrides concern for the other. The other, the object, may come to enjoy the sexual contact but frequently is aware it is not appropriate. The other comes to feel shame, disgust, and guilt with the realisation of what has happened. But sexual contact is addictive once an individual has been sexually aroused, so it is not surprising the activity continues despite reluctance. Rewards make it even harder to break free. Is it any wonder it is hard to recognise this abuse and exploitation and to have the courage to try and do something about it? Sexual abuse can lead to splitting and denial. The internal world becomes damaged and depleted. There is often a bubble of unprocessed experience that has not been remembered, digested, or integrated. Emotions can be projected or lost so deeply in the unconscious that they are not known. Aspects of this damage may present as post-traumatic disorder, emotional flatness, depression or despair, loss of intellectual capacity, panic attacks, and difficult relationships.

Where there is exploitation, then the damage is more profound. Irving Kaufman, in his book on abuse, wrote about Soul Murder, where there is exploitation, Kaufman (1989). This is much worse. Sexual abuse can split the internal world into part objects. Exploitation fragments the internal world and lays it bare, like a nuclear winter. The individual becomes dominated by pleasure and unpleasure, dominated by sensations. So thought or reflection is lost. Any sense of morality or decency can disappear. Instant gratification is desired; why wait? This can lead to a ruthlessness in gaining what the self wants and a disregard for others. Friendships are transitory and goal directed, for example, introducing others to the exploiting adults for their own rewards. Individual victims become hard and street wise. They grow a shell that is pretty impermeable. Sex and sexual gratification dominate their thinking. Aroused, their bodies seem to crave sexual satisfaction alongside any drugs or alcohol addictions that have been encouraged. The material benefits are also valued. They confer status within their peer group, and since many of the victims are from vulnerable and deprived situations, this is also important.

When the shell does crack, when the individual sees the depravity or is discarded having grown up a little, then it is heartbreaking to witness. There is fear and terror if they start to talk about what has happened to them. They fear being tracked down and found, then punished, or even destroyed. This dread and panic make reaching them very difficult. They can appear to go crazy or psychotic, but this is usually pseudo-psychosis. Where there is post-traumatic stress, the flashbacks and re-experiencing can be so vivid that others think they are out of touch with reality. In a way, they are but it is part of the trauma rather than a true psychotic illness. But some do briefly become properly psychotic. In this state, many need residential or inpatient placement. It seems that the trauma and stresses are of such intensity that some individuals lose contact with reality. They may need a safe place or medication or both to recover. Perhaps they were innately more vulnerable. What underlies all this is deep and intense desperation. They feel destroyed and finished, that their life is ruined, and death is the only option. They are very much at risk of suicide.

Both sexual abuse and sexual exploitation can respond to help and treatment. People who have been abused and exploited need to be kept safe from themselves and possible pursuers. The emotional storms are intense, violent anger at themselves, at others, and at those trying to keep them safe. The distress, weeping unconsolably, and begging for comfort but also sex and substances can be hard to manage. It is not easy to know when to encourage the individual to talk and when to help them rediscover their humanity to focus on other things. If there are relatives or committed foster carers, then their involvement can be helpful. When guilt and shame finally emerge, however, such contacts can be purgatorial, just too much for the individual.

Sexual abuse does seem to be quite common. Sexual exploitation is more frequent than recognised. Its consequence is untold damage to individuals, families, and communities.

Note

1 The NHS is the UK National Health Service

References

Butler-Sloss, E. 1988. *Report of the Inquiry into Child Abuse in Cleveland*. London, Department of Health.
Kaufman, I. 1989. *Soul Murder*, in Shengold M. D. (eds) *The Effects of Childhood Abuse and Deprivation*. Connecticut and London: Yale University Press.

11

CHILD SEXUAL EXPLOITATION IN A REFUGEE CONTEXT

The assault on protection

Krisna Catsaras

Introduction

This chapter offers some observations on child sexual exploitation in a refugee context from psychoanalytic and systems-psychodynamics perspectives. These observations are partially derived from the experience of a UK-based psychoanalytically oriented supervisory group, "Therapeutic Support Network: Lesvos", established to support a team of Greek psychologists working for a charity ("Ray of Hope" 🔲) offering shelter and psychosocial support to unaccompanied refugee children in Lesvos, Greece. The project lasted two years between September 2019 and October 2021.

The chapter will aim to contextualise child sexual exploitation as emerging in more widely degraded systems and abusive environments. It will understand immediate instances of abuse as stemming, in part, from destructive processes playing out at broader psychosocial levels, which drive the deterioration and dehumanisation of the contexts in which child sexual exploitation proliferates, but which also penetrate downwards, from a hostile social environment into individual psyches. This abuse will also be shown to be mirrored in the experience of the organisations and teams working with unaccompanied asylum-seeking children. They are, themselves, both embedded within and suffer the profoundly vexed national and transnational social and political conflicts which ultimately govern the macro responses to refugees and asylum seekers.

This is also to make the claim that the disturbing broader reality of child sexual exploitation cannot be simply collapsed and projected into accounts of individual perpetrators and victims only. Disaggregating acts of sexual abuse and sexual exploitation from the structural violence and social turmoil pervading their contexts are radically reductive, limiting culpability to individual actors.

DOI: 10.4324/9781003020370-11

Actively hostile policies, for example, which attack the needs of unaccompanied asylum-seeking children by undermining or destroying the structures that should protect and care for them in intensely unstable, dehumanised, and dangerous environments, or misrepresentation and exploitation of their precarious situations for political ends, are also profoundly implicated in the abuse of power that ultimately is child sexual exploitation.

Structure of the chapter

The chapter will culminate with a specific case example, the story of "Farid" ⌊OBJ⌋, a nine-year-old unaccompanied asylum-seeking child whose history of sexual exploitation reflected, with intense immediacy, these realities on the ground. It was the experience of the therapeutic support team, through both helping to process the historic reports of child abuse and child exploitation, and through engaging with current emerging safeguarding concerns in relation to the refugee children being sheltered and supported by "Ray of Hope", such as Farid, that it was not possible to fully comprehend these phenomena decontextualised from the turmoil in Lesvos and the macro events that were affecting the refugee situation in the Eastern Mediterranean. To some degree, it was possible to correlate the increasing child sexual exploitation concerns that we "witnessed" through our supervisory support with the evident deterioration in the broader socio-political context.

This chapter is therefore structured to mirror the cascade of these processes, starting at more generalised macro levels, and moving downwards in scale, becoming more immediate, localised, and "humanised". It will begin with a glance at some of the research which describes the desperate plight and unmet needs of unaccompanied asylum-seeking children and the failures, or "blind spots", of the child protection systems which are meant to protect them. In relation to the latter, much research focuses on the inadequacies and under-development of legal and administrative structures and child welfare systems. The shortcomings in the protection of unaccompanied asylum-seeking children are often accounted for, predominantly, as stemming from a lack of planning, skills, and resources; the passive result of a lack of coordination and thought, or, at worst, indifference. However, the lacunae in child protection also need to be understood, in part, as the outcome of destructive political and psychosocial processes, the outcome of mobilised and motivated attacks on this population, both conscious and unconscious. Examples of the literature that focuses on the hostile socio-political forces that drive these failures will, therefore, also be touched on.

The next section will then explore some of the specific aspects of the predicament of asylum-seeking children that make them vulnerable to exploitation, as well as the contextual dynamics at pressurised and politicised national borders, from broadly psychoanalytic and systems-psychodynamics perspectives. These processes are highly volatile, undermining efforts to build protective systems and establish stable norms for the care and well-being of asylum-seeking children. They are also invariably traumatogenic processes for everyone coming into any real and sustained contact with them. These forces contribute to a destructive "turning of a blind eye", both individual and collective. A psychoanalytic account of the processes involved in "turning a blind eye" forms a central conceptual framework for understanding the "passive" collusion of the human systems that are present and are meant to take responsibility for the care and protection of children whilst there is abuse in plain sight.

The chapter will then turn to a more experience-near account of the presence of these dynamics through the "Therapeutic Support Network: Lesvos" project and the impact they had on all levels of the work. Space will be made in this section to first give an overview of the geopolitical context and historical events at the time, moving from the broader situation to the regional location and then the organisation we worked with, to give a sense of the violation and exploitation of the total environment. This was the context in which Farid's story emerged.

The chapter will conclude with what might be drawn from this experience, including an outline of what could be considered a core psychological and ethical conflict experienced by professionals working in these environments. It will also touch on the significance and value of psychoanalytic supervision (within a systems-psychodynamics perspective) as an attempt to cast "an ethical eye" (when adequately self-reflective and within limits, and subject to its own ambivalence, lapses, and failures, and also subject to the forces and pressures discussed throughout this chapter) as a counterforce to the "turning of a blind eye".

The lack of child protection: Hostile environments

According to an IFRC (International Federation of Red Cross and Red Crescent Societies) report, published shortly before the start of the project but still pertinent at the time of writing, "the number of children on the move, including those travelling alone, has grown substantially and alarmingly in the past decade. There is compelling evidence that a very large proportion of them are exposed to sexual and gender-based violence on their journeys". Furthermore, protecting unaccompanied children along their entire migratory route from these risks, and ensuring access to needed services, "is a 'blind spot' for many governments and humanitarian organizations" (IFRC, 2018, p. 8). The report continues, citing research, that "regardless of the path taken … when children resort to unsafe routes, and are traveling without the protection of caring adults, they are at significantly increased risk of suffering sexual and gender-based violence by ill-intentioned smugglers and other unscrupulous actors, being sold into labour or sex exploitation by traffickers or forced into 'survival sex' to gain passage, shelter, sustenance or money for onward journeys" (ibid. p. 14).

Freccero et al (2017), in their review of recent literature on trafficking and exploitation in humanitarian settings, cite a number of risk factors that exacerbate these problems. These include "the erosion of the rule of law, lack of legal status, restrictions on movement, and the development of criminal networks to target new victims such as refugees. A lack of employment opportunities, inadequate access to protection and support services, insufficient and inequitable distribution of food and aid, and a loss of family and community support mechanisms also increase vulnerability to exploitation and abuse" (p. 3).

Digidiki and Bhabha (2018) highlight the exposure of these children due to "the absence of safe and legal paths to appropriate migration destinations, the impossibility of returning home to oppressive and harmful environments and the daily exposure to unsatisfactory, sometimes inhumane, living conditions inside migrant facilities" (p. 114). They also note a number of systemic failures in both government and non-government responses to the children's needs. "Among the most important are the absence of an integrated child protection system that spans national and local jurisdictions, the failure of existing child welfare systems to classify unaccompanied migrant children as a distinct and unique population requiring immediate attention and care irrespective of migration status, and the lack of properly trained and qualified staff to work with this uniquely vulnerable population". They concluded "that the current situation is evidence not of a migration crisis per se, but of a crisis in child protection" (ibid, p. 114).

Unaccompanied asylum-seeking children fall between the cracks in the system and get trapped there, "leading to an intensification of precarity", an increasingly common concept which generally refers to "a context of uncertainty, exploitation, restriction, and a status that is impermanent" (Barn op. cit, p. 2). Asylum-seeking children face increased precarity despite the obligations nations face under the United Nations Convention on the Rights of the Child, UNCRC (1989), of which almost every country in the world is a signatory. This commits them to the protection of the rights of all children, including refugee children (particularly in relation to Article 2 on non-discrimination). Though "a failure to afford adequate protections" (ibid, p. 3) is self-evident, the predicament of these children is one of "politically induced precariousness" which results in "real or symbolic violence" (Chase, 2020, p. 440).

There is a dissonance or split in political and social values, and a denial or disavowal of the consequences. As Barn et al note, it would appear that in dealing with the protection needs of unaccompanied asylum-seeking children, "European governments face the challenge of how to comply with their international and humanitarian obligations at a time when their overall concerns have shifted towards tougher immigration policies and stricter border control to curb unauthorised immigration". Furthermore, "although the processes of integration and mobility remain key challenges for nation-states, increasingly, we are witnessing the contradictions between liberal democratic espousals of freedom and equality and the reality of exclusionary immigration policies" (2021, pp. 1–2).

This is reinforced by processes through which those most in need become discredited and dehumanised. Ineffective protection policies are further undermined by exposure to a broader attitude of "victimisation and criminalisation" (Ayotte, 2000) towards asylum-seeking children across Europe. There is a "culture of disbelief and suspicion" (House of Lords, 2016) about their ages, stories, and motives. Barn et al, referencing Jacqueline Bhabha (2014), an expert in international law, migration, and children's rights, identify the tensions which exist between asylum advocacy and human rights in a context where migration from the Global South is "viewed with heightened suspicion and hostility" (2021, p. 3).

The hostile environment that refugee children face means that the failures in protection are not limited to their migration journeys. Indeed, returning to the IFRC report cited earlier, "the risks of sexual and gender-based violence do not abate once arriving in a second or third country ... New forms of exploitation and abuse manifest where protective services are overstretched or non-existent in places where migrant children land" (IFRC, 2018, p. 16). This has been the case across Europe. For example, they cite a UNICEF report which found that threats to their safety "have been incessant in countries like France, where children have struggled to benefit from protection mechanisms" (ibid. p. 30). "Similar studies in the UK have reached similar conclusions" (ibid, p. 17). This chapter draws from the experience of work in the Greek context, in which "a long list of factors ... have increased the chances of unaccompanied children falling victim to sexual violence, including shortages of living spaces ... that force children to cohabitate with adults in crowded settings, and a general lack of safety and security at the facilities, including poor lighting. The lack of safe housing options has led many unaccompanied migrant children in Greece to move to informal encampments where they are exposed to an even greater range of risks, including, for boys, being sexually abused and exploited by older men for money" (ibid, pp. 16–17).

"Borderline space": Contextual social and psychological dynamics of asylum-seeking children's experience

Physically, legally, and psychosocially unprotected spaces can facilitate the proliferation of child sexual exploitation. The spaces that forced migrant populations occupy, and get caught in, are often at the "borderlines", in various forms of "no man's land" and "buffer zones". These are unstable, conflicted, and highly volatile spaces at all levels of analysis: whether politically, socially, or interpersonally. The perception and understanding of these zones are prone to distortion and confusion, and the affects connected to them subject to intense amplification. Unpredictable and uncontained chronic volatility can disrupt and undermine personal, familial, and social norms, throwing their protective functions into disarray, and exposing the most vulnerable to exploitation. Under intense, disorienting pressures, these zones can become socially and psychologically collapsed and regressed spaces. The worst impulses can become uncontained and unmediated, no longer inhibited by these norms. It is well understood that such spaces are magnets for individuals and gangs seeking to exploit them.

Unaccompanied asylum-seeking children have particular psychological vulnerabilities to this exploitation. The refugee predicament is often understood through a trauma narrative, though there is some debate around this. Although still recognising that their histories are often profoundly traumatic, these debates are partly driven by concerns around the stigmatisation and victimisation of refugees and the limiting perceptions of them through such frameworks. But what then could be said to be the essential characteristics of the unaccompanied refugee child's predicament? Perhaps most definitively, they have lost both their homes and the protection of their parents or other adult figures responsible for their care. Papadopoulos (2002) notes that "… loss of home is the only condition that all refugees share, not trauma. Refugees are defined not as a group of people exhibiting any specific psychological condition but merely as people who have lost their home" (p. 9). Alongside this very real homelessness is a simultaneous psychic "un-housing". Papadopoulos goes on to explore the multifaceted meanings of "home" and the loss of secure belonging in a state of homelessness, and the frustrated yearning of what he calls "nostalgic disorientation".

For unaccompanied children, there is this further essential dimension in their experience of parentless-ness, compounding the loss of a basic sense of safety and security with disrupted attachments and the frustration of basic psychological needs. Separated from parents and families, they have certainly faced significant developmental trauma, at a bare minimum: a degree of premature and traumatic separation; a breaking of bonds. The yearning for home is simultaneously also the cry of unmet dependency needs. The ensuing lack of protection and nurture, and access to resources, both physical and psychological, leaves them vulnerable to abuse and the exploitation of these dependency needs.

More intra-psychically, depending on a child's developmental history, there may be a deterioration of the psychological structures that develop in childhood. From a psychoanalytic perspective, this might include an undermining of oedipal developments including what has previously been internalised of the experience of "good parents".[1] These form both a sense of basic trust and internal security, but, as importantly in this context, also help the modulation and socialisation of basic drives and impulses (both sexual and aggressive). The development of capacities for managing these is dependent on parenting. Without responsible parents helping the management of socially appropriate interpersonal behaviour, including psychological boundaries around sexuality and aggression, and without having developed a mature sense of personal agency (in any meaningful way and at a real depth of personality), children are more vulnerable to serious transgressions in the absence of parental protection and guidance. Returning to a broader, more systemic perspective, it is also the broader child protection "system" around refugees that lacks this "parenting function" and sense of "parental" responsibility to care for these children. The destruction of social protective systems for unaccompanied children is an attack on their dependency.

Unaccompanied asylum-seeking children are also crossing borders and are often caught up in the terrain around them. What is it about the "psychic geography" of borders that can create such unstable spaces psychologically and psychosocially? Borders, as with boundaries, can have necessary protective aspects. Both can provide often negotiable "limits" that require and provide regulation. This chapter will not argue against the necessity or inevitability of borders and boundaries. When they are functioning well, they provide aspects of the conditions for exchange and communication, reception, various forms of relationship, and interdependence. However, when subject to paranoia, extreme threat, or breakdown, they can become dangerous. Borders can then become absolute schismatic lines that can both generate and attract intense anxieties and conflict. These intense anxieties can then stimulate an equally intense need for their control. The greater the anxiety, the more rigid and concrete this need can become. Any sense of threat and instability from one side of a boundary can also be projected to the other, thus reinforcing this need even further.

Ultimately, though they are partially generated by and map onto geographical space, borders are also human constructs brought into being, and sustained, psychologically and socially. The psychological pressure territorial borders generate contributes to a collapse from more open, expansive, and receptive three-dimensional mental states to two-dimensional cartographies in the mind, where a line is drawn to separate inside and outside, this side and that, in-groups from out-groups: multi-dimensional complexities reduced and divided into binaries. As such, they can quickly become frontiers of tension and violence.

In psychoanalytic terms, they are both the source and target of intense splitting and projection and subject to more rudimentary and self-protecting states of mind, at the expense of a relationship with the other, or the other's survival altogether. Intense anxieties around the multiple meanings of contact and, with it, the threat of the transgression of boundaries can be easily and rapidly mobilised. This does not always need to depend on a sense of immediacy or proximity. They can be experienced either near geographical and national borders or projected onto them from afar.

Based on perennial human concerns, they can usually be gathered into three sets of interconnected anxieties: security anxieties (including the threat of invasion and disease); cultural anxieties (threats to identity and ways of life); and resource anxieties (whether through theft, competition, or exploitation of those resources). A quick look at the content of right-wing European media during the "refugee crisis" reveals how they can become amplified, distorted, and weaponised (Berry et al, 2015). Cartoons, articles, and images depict terrorists, floods, and pests; fears of the "Islamification of Europe"; the blaming of refugees for rises in crime, exploitation of the welfare state, or the taking away of employment opportunities for nationals. The greater the degree of anxiety, the more "othered" and then dehumanised those people onto whom these anxieties are projected become, and the more implicitly (and sometimes explicitly) racialised the discourse. One's own individual and collective unwanted aspects can also be projected onto the "other". The ensuing sense of threat coming from the "other" often obscures how terrifying and dangerous contact with "us" can be for those fleeing other dangers.

"Turning a blind eye"

The tendency, then, is to "turn a blind eye" to this distress. Steiner (1985) returns to Sophocles' tragedy "Oedipus Rex" for a psychoanalytic exploration of this phenomenon, whereby disavowal is the central concern: paradoxically being aware and unaware of a disturbing reality at the same time. It is worth taking a moment to give a summary of Steiner's account. Oedipus, as Steiner reminds his reader, blinds himself at the climax of the play in a moment of "truly heroic acknowledgement" when he fully faces and avows the truth of his situation: the tragic and traumatic realisation that he has killed his father and slept with his mother. This, at least, is the traditional interpretation of the play. However, Steiner suggests that there is a second current of intrigue in the play, happening *simultaneously* alongside this first one, which is open to an alternative interpretation. He argues that, as the clues were there from the beginning, all the main characters, including Oedipus and the chorus, must have been aware of Oedipus' identity and realised that he had committed parricide and incest at much, much earlier points in the play, not just towards the end. However, they all participate in some degree of denial and disavowal throughout, which Steiner uses the term "turning a blind eye" to describe. Furthermore, Steiner argues, the clues are all there for a discerning audience or reader to be aware of also. If this is the case, the audience also participates at some level in this "turning of a blind eye" in seeing only the former interpretation (the tragic realisation) and not the secondary one (they knew, at some level, all along). At the heart of disavowal is a traumatic event beyond the mind's capacity for containment. At the same time, the cost of disavowal of this knowledge includes our "passive" collusion and "ignorant" participation.

It is important to recognise that this collapse into passivity follows contact with what is experienced as an impossible trauma, seemingly irreparable and unforgivable, which we feel powerless to address. However, there is a risk of denying the more violent and *active* impulses which seek to destroy both the awareness of this reality and those who represent it also. The vulnerability of the refugee situation is routinely blanked out. Actively hostile processes, xenophobic and racialised, are mobilised and reinforce this non-recognition: denying the reality of their predicament or seeking their annihilation altogether. The knowledge that what is most disturbing lives "within" us is also destroyed, projected as it is onto the "other", but it keeps returning to haunt us. The "perpetrators" of the systemic abuse explored in this chapter may initially seem "foreign" but are also found to operate in the liminal spaces on "our" borders. Most disturbing is the realisation that they operate "within": within our borders, within the abusive, neglectful, and exploitative practices of a hostile system, and within spaces that are not "other", including our own minds. If the system is actively unprotective or hostile, it is one in which we are all implicated when collectively "turning a blind eye".

Historical/geopolitical context

The project undertaken in partnership with "Ray of Hope" took place during a period of intense geopolitical stress which, from a Eurocentric perspective, was playing out at the Greek border and "beyond". 2015 was the start of a significant increase in the movement of refugees and asylum-seekers towards Europe, when 1.3 million people came towards the continent to request asylum that year. In addition to ongoing conflicts elsewhere, the surge was in large part due to the wars and ensuing crises in Syria, Iraq, and Afghanistan, as well as terrorist insurgencies and chronic human rights abuses in other countries. The largest numbers initially came via the "southern Mediterranean route" (mainly Italy), but by the end of 2015, 80% were crossing the Turkish-Greek border, either via the mainland or the Aegean Sea. Numbers remained very high but gradually reduced towards the end of 2015, and then significantly reduced following the implementation of the infamous "EU-Turkey deal", signed in March 2016. The policy, initially intended to be temporary, has been catastrophic for asylum seekers who continue to be caught up in the legal and administrative vacuum it created.

Large numbers became immobilised and trapped in borderline spaces, such as the Greek island of Lesvos, and in the infamous Moria refugee camp, which will be described below. Living conditions became increasingly dehumanised, bringing about a significant deterioration in both physical and mental health. Tensions in these spaces became ever more heightened, both by specific events and chronic strain, and eventually became explosive. The account below starts at a macro-level, from which this strain cascaded downwards into increasingly pressurised and strained communities and organisations, which became more fragmented, conflicted, and atomised.

At the same time, there was a reneging of responsibility by those in authority in relation to the crisis, and a reciprocal sense of abandonment in those dependent on them, as well as a loss of faith in leadership: Greece experienced a lack of solidarity from the EU; the island of Lesvos felt abandoned by mainland Greece; NGOs on Lesvos faced increasing levels of hostility from aspects of the local community; frontline NGO workers felt unprotected and unsupported by their managers. This cascading sense of systemic abandonment was finally acted out on unaccompanied children, repeating and mirroring their histories of profound separation and loss, and own sense of abandonment. What limited systems of care and protection for unaccompanied children there were put under further pressures and prone to dysfunction and breakdown or actively targeted and dismantled. Asylum seekers, rather than finding refuge, safety, and containment in the positive sense, became themselves, as they so often are, receptacles of projected anxiety and hostility.

During this period of chronic turmoil and heightened social anxiety, stoked, and amplified as ever by right-wing media, there was a shift towards more right-wing politics in Greece, as elsewhere. An initially fairly receptive and humanitarian public response swung towards a hostile and securitised one. There were increasing reports of "pushbacks" (possibly a euphemism for much worse human rights violations) of asylum-seekers, both by land and sea. Mitsotakis, leader of the centre-right "New Democracy" party, became prime minister in July 2019, taking power from left-wing Syriza. However, there were several members of New Democracy with affiliations to the far right who were put in positions of power. The Greek government then took a hard-line stance. An Amnesty International report from June 2021, following up an original report in 2013 which had already raised concerns about the "pushbacks" of refugees and migrants, stated that Greece was "still violently and illegally returning people to Turkey, in contravention of their human rights obligations under EU and international law". Amnesty described these pushbacks as having become the "de facto policy of Greek border control" under Mitsotakis's government and stated that this was actively supported by Frontex, the EU's border agency. Greece had very much become the gatekeeper of "Fortress Europe".

Local and national narratives quickly grew in response to the extraordinary impact of large numbers of asylum-seekers on the shores of Greece. Initially, the quality of "filoxenia", something akin to hospitality as a virtue, the love of strangers, was heralded. Caring, open receptivity was foregrounded. Close behind or underneath was its antithesis, which soon came to the fore – hardened borders, hostility, and rejection. This oscillation made itself visible in the public narrative in manifold ways. I remember landing in Athens airport on the way to Lesvos to meet "Ray of Hope's" psychology teams at an earlier stage of the project and walking past a series of adverts for a famous whisky brand on the travelator. The advertising campaign was using a series of portraits of Greek fishermen who had saved the lives of asylum-seekers at sea. They had been nominated as potential Nobel prize winners. Just a year later, on a follow-up visit to the teams and the camps, the winds of public opinion were blowing in the opposite direction. As I walked along the same travelator, the whisky brand ad campaign had changed, tapping this change of mood and attitude. In place of life-saving fishermen were images of the great northern "Wall" from the HBO series "Game of Thrones": a massive, frozen defence sealing out "the Wildlings" and other threats from beyond the borders of the kingdom it served to protect.

Lesvos and Moria refugee camp

"The world's deadliest border"[2] (Jones, 2017, p. 12) had become even more dangerous. Lying in this treacherous zone is the Greek island of Lesvos, already a strategic and geopolitical tension point at the border between Greece and Turkey. It was home to the Moria refugee camp, which had been very much foregrounded in the European media between 2015 and 2016 during what was deemed to be the height of the "refugee crisis". Until it was destroyed by a fire in September 2020, it was the largest refugee camp in Europe. As it spilt over into neighbouring olive groves, it grew into a tent city, with often makeshift shelters made from wooden pallets and tarpaulins. As with all such under-planned and under-resourced cramped and crowded living spaces, it was squalid and dehumanising. It was originally built to accommodate three thousand people. By summer 2020, it held 20,000 people, amongst whom were six to seven thousand children.

As well as a very real geographical site, Moria became a "place in the mind" and a striking example of a space that was projected into and then kept fenced and sealed off, so that anxieties could remain encapsulated there or even annihilated. With an ever-hardening stance, refugee camps, such as Moria, rather than being transitional spaces for temporarily sheltering vulnerable populations whilst solutions were sought, began to be envisioned as closed centres. Concerns were raised that they were, in effect, becoming detention centres, with the sense of something being caged off and "contained" at the expense of those human beings locked away. It is important to note the very different meanings of this sort of "containment" as restricting and limiting and trapping sources of anxiety, rather than containment in a psychoanalytic sense, which helps to process, make sense of, and ameliorate anxiety, and thus facilitate a capacity to think and reflect.

Lesvos had become a focal point, politically, socially, and in the eyes of the European media. As the number of asylum-seekers continued to rise, so did the influx of other players. Frontex ships lined the harbour. There was a build-up of police and other state forces. International humanitarian organisations also became a substantial and visible presence. Alongside more serious NGOs, a number of start-up organisations arrived on the island. Some of these added to the disorganisation and chaos and generated further unnecessary resentment. As the energy around the island grew, Lesvos became a magnet for increasingly polarised forces. Neo-Nazi groups came from across Europe and infiltrated the local community. In response, groups coming under the broad umbrella of "Antifa" arrived also. Before long, the sense of any middle ground had collapsed, and violence ensued.

There was a serious intensification of unrest from February 2020 onwards, which also provides both the contemporaneous context to the case example later below. As the chaos increased, so did concerns about child sexual abuse and exploitation in general across the supervisory work.

In early February 2020, hundreds of asylum seekers had converged on Mytilene, the island's capital, to protest about the horrendous conditions inside the overcrowded Moria refugee camp. As tensions escalated with aspects of the local community, the Greek government shipped in squads of riot police to the island. However, there were further riots at almost the same time against the arrival of construction teams with excavating machines who were to start building the new closed camps on Lesvos. Groups both hostile to the presence of asylum-seekers on the island on the one hand, and groups mobilised against the effective incarceration of refugees in these detention centres on the other, were for once united in this protest. Their protests were broken up with tear gas.

There was an ever-heightening general contextual dynamic of explosive rage, forceful oppression, and ever-increasing resentment towards the refugees and asylum seekers themselves. NGOs on the island also started suffering increased hostility from local groups. Aid workers' reports to various news outlets at the time included harassment, intimidation, and, in some cases, violence. Gangs of men were going into hotels and demanding to know whether any NGO workers were there. They were attacked in the street and their hire cars smashed up. Journalists, as witnesses to the situation, were also attacked, as were doctors working inside the Moria refugee camp. It was not long before the state also began to criminalise the presence of certain NGOs.

Just when the tensions in Lesvos seemed like they could not intensify further, changes in Turkish policy, driven by different factors but which may also have been cynically exploiting the situation, rocked the island further. Turkey's ongoing involvement in the civil war in Syria increased with a cross-border operation on 27th February 2020 into Idlib province, which led to the deaths of 33 Turkish soldiers and the next large influx of

Syrian refugees from that region into Turkey. On the next day, 28th February 2020, Turkey announced that it was unilaterally opening its borders to Greece to allow refugees and migrants seeking refuge to reach the European Union. However, this also timed with ongoing territorial border "disputes" between the two countries, connected with the discoveries of large reserves of hydrocarbons in the eastern Mediterranean, as well as increases in nationalist and expansionist sentiments globally. The change in policy could also, therefore, be seen as a result of the instrumental use and exploitation of refugees for geostrategic ends.

At the same time, the Covid pandemic had reached Europe. Unsurprisingly, it was quickly weaponised by right-wing media. Nationalists blamed migrants for the spread of Covid. Lesvos, as with all of Greece, was under strong lockdown measures, which also meant Moria. This was an extremely frightening time to be in an overcrowded refugee camp with next to no medical facilities or support. By May 2020, pandemic measures were being relaxed for the general population of Lesvos but were extended for migrants, and Moria remained under lockdown. On 2nd September 2020, in response to the first confirmed Covid case in the camp, the Greek government enforced a potentially harmful quarantine on all migrants and asylum seekers living there (Medicins Sans Frontières, 2022). Notis Mitarachi, the minister for migration, told local news that the coronavirus situation demonstrated the need for "closed and controlled" structures (Sto Nisi, 2020). The Migration ministry then released a further statement a couple of days later through which the plans to create closed structures on the islands of Lesvos and Chios were given renewed vigour. It was a very cynical approach, manipulating anxieties about the pandemic as an excuse to supplement further restrictions that were not justified from a public health point of view. A few days later, on 8th September 2020, a fire almost completely destroyed the camp. By then, its population had reduced to 12,000 asylum seekers. Most of the refugees were left homeless on the street. During protests demanding their evacuation Greek police once again fired tear gas at them.

As might be anticipated, the deteriorating conditions had a very serious impact on the well-being of refugees and asylum-seekers. An IRC report, from December 2020, citing data collated over the previous two and a half years on Lesvos, Samos, and Chios, the three Greek islands most impacted by the "refugee crisis", presented evidence of severe mental health conditions following "years of entrapment". As many as three out of four of the people the IRC had assisted through its mental health programme on the three islands reported one form of diagnostic mental health issue or another. Over the year outlined above (2020), there was a rise in the proportion of people disclosing psychotic symptoms, from one in seven to one in four. Disclosures of self-harm had increased by 66%. One in three people had contemplated suicide, whilst one in five reported having made attempts to take their lives.

Describing conditions in the camps as dangerous and inhumane, the IRC report stated that residents were still denied access to sufficient water, sanitation, shelter, and vital services such as healthcare, education, and legal assistance to process asylum claims. Lesvos was also cited as the island most often targeted by traffickers working along the Turkish coast. At the same time, alongside deterioration in mental health and living conditions, there were increased reports of exploitation and abuse.

"Ray of Hope" and "Therapeutic Support Network: Lesvos"

"Ray of Hope" was a locally based indigenous charity initially established to support marginalised and vulnerable groups in Lesvos and facilitate social integration. With the sudden influx of refugees and asylum-seekers into Lesvos in 2015, the charity rapidly grew, and its primary task evolved into a focus on refugee children, taking predominantly unaccompanied children from the refugee camps into nearby sheltered accommodation. At the point that our team began its engagement with them, "Ray of Hope" was supporting approximately 150 children, mainly adolescents. They were housed in six or seven "shelters", mainly houses in the island's capital, Mytilene. Space at the shelters was very cramped. The smaller shelters housed around fifteen to twenty young people, the largest up to around forty. Each shelter was staffed by a multi-disciplinary team including social workers, coordinators, care workers, and psychologists. There were also lawyers allocated to several shelters at a time who had responsibility for their asylum cases. The psychologists were given a broad remit providing a range of input that would fall under the broad umbrella of "psychosocial work".

We established our project, "Therapeutic Support Network: Lesvos", in autumn 2019. We were a UK-based team of child psychotherapists and group analysts, with experience of working with asylum-seeking children in the United Kingdom, and international NGO work in related fields, seeking to make a small supportive contribution in response to the "refugee crisis" in Greece. We sought, in a bespoke way, to come alongside a charity that was already doing direct work with unaccompanied asylum-seeking children, which met a number of criteria that would make us a good "fit".

"Ray of Hope" was established and domestic, meaning that it was home-grown with roots in the local community, allowing a greater sense of its relative permanence. It was more integrated locally and not a trans-national or international import. Given its sheltering of children in houses within the local community and outside of the camps, as well as its being staffed by Greek teams on initially longer-term contracts, rather than the rapid turnover of the well-known international agencies, whose staff often do time-limited "tours of duty", we hoped to build a durable relationship with this charity, and not a transient and disrupted one. Unaccompanied children frequently face cycles of disrupted relationships. There is often a high and rapid rate of turnover amongst staff working with them in these environments, thus repeating the experience of broken attachments. Organisations seeking to offer psychosocial and psychological support to refugee children can, therefore, sometimes unhelpfully mirror the population they are trying to serve. We hoped to build long-term relationships to provide a counterforce to this unhelpful dynamic.

When we began our work with "Ray of Hope", we understood that there had been high levels of "burnout" in the psychology teams and an increasingly rapid turnover of staff as a result. We hoped to help reduce this and, by doing so, help staff build longer-term connections with these children. Burnout in such circumstances is often conceptualised as the result of secondary trauma. Professionals working in these fields are working with people suffering high levels of trauma and loss, often communicated through intense states of rage and terror, grief, and despair. Working with asylum-seekers also often involves psychologically taxing experiences of chronic uncertainty. Asylum cases can often get stuck for many months. In Lesvos, it was not uncommon for asylum-seeking children to be awaiting decisions for up to two years, sometimes longer.

Though secondary trauma is a necessary aspect of any conceptualisation of burnout in this setting, it is incomplete. The focus is too often exclusively on the difficulties emerging "bottom up" rather than "top down": comprehending the psychological impact of working with traumatised and abused children whilst paying less attention to the traumatised organisations and systems in which this work is taking place. Low morale is a significant aspect of burnout and is often linked to a loss of faith in leadership, or increasing dissonance with what is felt to be an organisation's core values. However, in line with the argument throughout this chapter, this often occurs at macro levels and then percolates downwards. The psychologists working for "Ray of Hope" were working for an organisation that was itself frequently left unsupported, starved of funding, and attacked. From this perspective, the burnout we were being asked to help address was also caused by the trauma, abuse, and despair engendered by the wider system itself. And again, this was not just due to systemic disorganisation but by destructive efforts to actively dis-organise. A core part of our "offer", then, needed to include a more systems-psychodynamics approach to these issues and to include a more organisational perspective.

Our central provision was once weekly one-to-one individual psychoanalytic supervision and psychological support for all "Ray of Hope's" psychologists remotely via Zoom or Skype. From the start, we planned to help develop an otherwise lacking culture of regular analytic supervision in addition to their system of general line management. They also needed help processing the impact of the work. As they were relatively inexperienced, a further aspect of our remit was to help them develop their clinical capacities for individual and group work and broader psychosocial work. It also became quickly evident that the supervisory support helped them maintain their judgement in relation to ethical practice and their awareness of safeguarding concerns when under immense pressures, in collapsing environments, to give up or look away.

In addition, our team met regularly in pairs to process the experience from our end and then as a team once every four to six weeks. As the project lead, I also received fortnightly supervision from a systems-psychodynamics perspective. Each supervisor built a picture of the shelter in which their supervisee worked, including its individual members, the sub-groups amongst the young people, the inter-disciplinary dynamics amongst the staff, and each shelter's main concerns. In our team meetings, we tried to build a picture of emergent thematic concerns across the shelters, as well as gaining a sense of how the organisation was functioning as a whole. The plan was to then meet with "Ray of Hope's" management once every six to eight weeks also, to give feedback on these generalised themes, share our reflections on the systems-psychodynamics in their charity, and raise any concerns.

Initial contact with the "system" and the teams: A pervasive sense of exploitation and distrust

A systems-psychodynamics approach to consulting emphasises the value of reflecting on the initial experience of contact with an organisation, and the way it manages its boundaries. These moments can provide important information about the underlying anxieties and concerns which may be driving an organisation's functioning. At the same time, the way an organisation becomes structured may not only be to perform the primary tasks for which it exists but also to defend itself from the anxieties related to those tasks.

Although communication with "Ray of Hope's" senior management became more regular and robust over time, the first meeting on-site was held without them and with the psychology teams themselves. It would do a disservice to the charity to misrepresent the leadership's overall commitment, but this initial absence was perhaps a noteworthy enactment of a central, mostly unconscious, dynamic. The young psychologists communicated their feelings of being unprotected and unsupported. As this was explored, it deepened into a sense of neglect, abandonment, and overwhelm. For some the work was traumatic. Others felt abused and exploited. Several felt close to burnout or referred to colleagues who had left. They were exhausted and morale was low. Staff teams often reflect the groups with which they work, and the psychologists were no different. Emotional proximity and identification with the children in their care meant that they were, to some degree, in a parallel process which was useful to reflect on.

More widely, tension and distrust between Greece and the EU were also pervasive. Greece not only felt unsupported during the refugee crisis but had also been suffering the fallout of a financial crisis that had started in 2009, and which led to the longest recession of any advanced mixed economy to date. There were intense social and political anxieties that the vulnerability of the Greek state was leaving it open to predatorial abuse by stronger EU economies, whilst social discourse was saturated with a combination of shame, anger, and resignation in the face of widespread corruption. The Greek people had suffered serious financial hardship due to harsh and protracted austerity measures, including brutal public sector cuts. The cost of living was rapidly increasing whilst salaries had plummeted. There was massive unemployment, especially amongst young people. Reciprocal themes of being under-resourced whilst experiencing financial exploitation ran through this early meeting. The organisation itself was frequently starved of funding. Promised resources did not come through and the psychologists could, in turn, go months without being paid. Being financially dependent on the charity meant that this was experienced as a cruel, humiliating, and perverse response to their own dependency needs.

However, several members of the team were also troubled by their own motives – were they working with unaccompanied children because it was an opportunity to develop their careers? Were they doing it for the money? There was a sense of confusion about who was exploiting whom. Towards the end of the first meeting, I was also challenged on our motives. What was in it for us? Who was paying us? Were we making a business out of the refugee crisis? They reminded me of the cynical exploitation of refugees who had drowned in the Aegean having been sold fake lifejackets by traffickers. Did we not realise that the whole refugee situation was big business, an industry? It is an uncomfortable truth also that there is a history of exploitation by the staff of various agencies supposedly deployed for protective purposes in humanitarian settings.[3]

This powerful experience at the organisation's boundary placed us in immediate contact with an environment of abuse and exploitation. Some of the signatures of the traumatic betrayal of dependency needs, including a deep cynicism and a sense of ethical disorientation, were evident. There was a fragile and undermined sense of the "good": of benign motives, trust, and dependability. Indeed, in our approach to the organisation, as well as being welcomed and seen to be offering a potentially valuable resource, there was a worry that we were also intending to predatorially feed off the refugee situation and develop a parasitical relationship with the charity. At its most unconscious, this perhaps included a reversal and exploitation of the earliest feeding relationship, symbolically preying on and exploiting their most vulnerable and infantile aspects during a period of maximal dependency. Together with recognising these sorts of anxieties, it was important to work with the ways they blended into more socio-political concerns, though these could sometimes be just as unconscious. For example, that we were patronising northern Europeans, remote but judgmental, and colonial in intent. We were, after all, most of the time thousands of miles away on our own island post-Brexit, turning away the relatively small numbers of asylum-seekers reaching our shores. We could keep our hands clean whilst allowing our southern European counterparts to do the dirty work.

In reality, we were a small voluntary team working unpaid. In retrospect, amongst other reasons, this may have partially been a way to defend ourselves against anxieties about exploitation, a way to hold onto a sense of the "good" in ourselves in a deeply ambivalent space. To sustain our involvement, we may have unconsciously needed to fend off the apprehension of unbearable guilt and shame inevitable in this space, as will be returned to later.

It was only after some months that these anxieties and dynamics around exploitation entered the real core of our supervisory work. However, as the contextual situation deteriorated, there were two related phenomena that did become more pronounced in supervision. The first was that incidents of child sexual exploitation, initially reported as being afar, became ever nearer and immediate: closer and closer to the shelters. Alarming stories of abuse initially related to the infiltration of other charities on the mainland. Soon, we heard of abuses in the extended networks of the young people in the shelters but located in the camps on the island. A little while later, this was taking place in closer proximity to the shelters in town. There was an uncanny sense of dread that this contact was coming closer, and it was not long before we were hearing reports involving children in the charity's care. There is a serious question as to whether this may have been happening all along inside the shelters, but that supervisory support helped make things clearer eyed. In a sense, getting increasingly in touch with these disturbing issues also brings them "inside" and no longer projected "outside". Was it a case of the abuse and exploitation getting deeper into the system as the environment deteriorated, or the development of a deeper and more distressing awareness of what was already there? Of course, these possibilities are not mutually exclusive.

The second simultaneous and related concern was in relation to various reports of troubling transgressions in professional boundaries between staff and young asylum seekers, alongside a slippage of perspective on other norms. Again, these were initially reported to be at a distance to the charity and its shelters. We heard of a young female social worker in another charity who was sacked following "an inappropriate relationship" with an unaccompanied male asylum seeker, though the psychologists thought that he was probably denying his real age and was in his early 20s, as she was, and therefore not a minor. Several of "Ray of Hope's" psychologists felt that there was something "othering" in holding a professional role in relation to the young people in their care. In an otherwise hostile environment, they felt that they should be more like their friends. After all, many of them were not all that much older than the late adolescents they were working with. The thought that these children needed them to maintain a boundaried professional role with a quasi-parental authority was undermined by an anxiety that this meant the exercise of a racialised power differential. It was as if to hold a boundary was to align oneself with the xenophobic hostility that was saturating the environment. At the same time, this was also perhaps due to feeling inadequate in their roles as a young and inexperienced team. Whatever the underlying anxieties, there were signs of a collapse in the sense of generational difference, risking a transgression of sexual boundaries and a potential abuse of power. What needed to be recognised also was the denied unconscious hostility in the seduction of a young person in a position of dependency. These issues were picked up by our team and helped maintain a normative expectation around professional boundaries and what the children needed from them as psychologists.

At the same time, there were indeed signs of racialised resentment and hostility towards the children within the charity's teams, but usually held and expressed by individuals amongst the 24-hour care staff. They were usually more deeply connected with the local community, which had suffered the most intense consequences of receiving tens of thousands of asylum seekers on their island and been left relatively unaided. They also had the most contact with the children. This is not, however, to justify the comments drawing on barely disguised prejudicial stereotypes of the children's various ethnicities or the sporadic acts of physical intimidation, both of which increased in periods when tensions were amplified on the island. These were reported back to management, and the psychologists were supported to seriously challenge these enactments and to reflect on what was happening – including most painfully in themselves. More serious breaches were dealt with through a disciplinary procedure, and some staff members were sacked. However, as with much of their experience, it was exhausting to maintain a struggle against these destructive processes.

"Farid"

Three quarters of the young people in "Ray of Hope's" care were adolescents. However, Farid's case was an example of the exploitation of one of the much younger children. An example of a child of any age could give a sense of how these dynamics entered individual cases. Farid and his younger sister "Amal" had been taken from Moria camp and brought to the shelters shortly ahead of some of the events above in January 2020. He was a nine-year-old Kurdish-Iraqi boy who had become separated from his parents when the boat they were being smuggled on from Turkey to Lesvos had sunk a year or so prior. Their whereabouts were unknown, and it is possible they had drowned. Farid had been "adopted" in Moria camp, and it took some time for professionals working with him to understand that the adults claiming responsibility for him were not his parents. It was realised alarmingly late that he was being routinely sexually abused and exploited. He was being pimped for money and rewarded with food and shelter. It is unclear whether his sister suffered similar treatment, though she did not later demonstrate the same hallmark behaviours as Farid.

Farid was initially in a shelter for younger children. When his case was first brought to supervision, this history was obscure. There was some knowledge held somewhere, but accounts were vague. Instead, he had come quickly on the radar due to his alarming behaviour. This began with his going to the toilet in inappropriate places (defecating in the small garden of the shelter), exposing himself to other children, and asking to touch their genitals. Staff understandably became alarmed by the risk he posed to other young children. However, there was a sense in which no-one really wanted to know what had happened to Farid. Though only nine years old, he could only be thought of as a perpetrator. They couldn't manage him within the house. They felt that no amount of observation or vigilance could keep the other children safe. A problem had arisen which needed to be evacuated. However, the charity's resources were extremely stretched and limited. Farid's case was lost in a backlog of asylum cases, and he was trapped on Lesvos. There were no equivalent charities on the island who could take care of him. They were either operating inside the camps or had been closed down. "Ray of Hope" itself was already in "survival mode", unsure how long funding would last or whether they would also be forced to close under new government policies. The only alternative provision available to the charity was to move him to one of the shelters for older adolescent boys.

It was not long before Farid was at the centre of a concern about sexual exploitation in that shelter also. He would "disappear" and be found in one of the shared rooms for the older boys. He seemed to be supplied with cans of fizzy drink and chocolates. Staff became very uncomfortable but were unable to identify what was happening or to articulate why they were so anxious about him. Concerns were flagged with management, and he was moved to another shelter … and then another.

Defensive manoeuvres against knowing about the sexual abuse and exploitation had taken on a different form once they had crossed the boundary into the shelters themselves. There was a form of group disavowal, or "turning a blind eye" at an organisational level. The problem was tackled by trying to move Farid, for a period the child in whom almost all concern about sexual exploitation was located, from one shelter to another, as if this would address the issue. When Farid was moved, the team at the shelter from which he was moved was quickly relieved, as if child sexual abuse and exploitation were no longer their concern. The new shelter would initially turn away from the problem and then would get highly anxious about Farid's manifest behaviour before he was moved on. In this way, concerns about sexual abuse and exploitation would be isolated in different shelters at different times, but there was never a sense of the concern being held across the team in a unified way.

Indeed, the psychology team itself was becoming fragmented, with increasing degrees of non-attendance at their weekly team meetings. It was as if unity would mean the integration of awareness and thinking across the teams, taking on collective responsibility, and therefore also the pain of shared guilt. Instead, cooperation and communication between the shelters kept being interrupted or discontinued, inhibited also by intense underlying shame. The disturbance was thus passed around and never held onto.

The denial was then intensified by a further disavowal of what had previously come into awareness. For example, supervisees in contact with these concerns through supervision would later collapse, exhausted, into "we don't know". There was a sincere uncertainty about whether certain exploitative sexual behaviour had taken place. "We don't know", however, also began to elide with a passive surrender – into giving up knowing. The level of risk was such that more ordinarily some form of action should have been taken, whether or not there was absolute certainty. Action based on awareness was routinely replaced by a stultifying doubt that was heavily incentivised by the wish not to know and relieve oneself of guilt and responsibility. However, ultimately, there was a sense of powerlessness and dread that they were unable to protect Farid, nor could they consistently sustain the protection of other children. There were simply no other sources of reliable support or child protection to turn to. They had to manage as best they could in the shelters.

Our supervision offered a "look" at what was going on, but this meant at times that it was felt to be persecutory and unwelcome. The psychologists held the disavowed awareness of what was happening but also experienced a terrifying moral culpability for having known what was going on when it came more clearly into the light. These dynamics were then reiterated in our team also as we were put in and out of touch in turn through our connections in supervision with different shelters. Our team also became alarmed and, at times, fragmented. Were we colluding with a charity in which abuse and exploitation were taking place? Were we turning a blind eye? We also experienced intense persecutory guilt whilst also encountering the reality that there were simply no authorities to report to or turn to beyond the charity who could themselves step in to protect the children. We, too, were left in a void without "parental" guidance and protection. The more this reality became apparent, the more our team began to split around these issues. The paranoid anxiety started to take over the team that we were doing something very wrong remaining involved. Who could we consult, beyond our team and our own supervision, to check our bearings? In an attempt to manage these anxieties, we consulted the ethical board of our governing organisation.

The board's view was that we were not in breach of any ethical guidelines, and they were deeply sympathetic to our project. However, there were no guidelines because we were in a space across borders without jurisdiction and an over-arching child protection framework.

It was only through attempting to work through these anxieties together in our team meetings that we could begin to integrate our perspectives and try to develop an overview. We were able to recognise that one aspect of this was that we were mirroring what was happening across the charity, though we had the luxury of a comfortable distance to become aware of this. All we could then offer was our understanding of what we thought was happening and facilitate greater communication and cooperation between the psychologists and their teams, as well as provide a "thinking space" for them to mobilise as much protective capacity and normative expectations within the shelters as possible.

In Farid's case, this led to a decision to reinstate regular group meetings with the adolescent boys in the shelter and a period of direct individual work between Farid and one of the psychologists, "Eleni", with whom he had already begun to build a more trusting relationship, under supervision. In their very first session, Farid picked up a pen and some paper and drew a picture of an erect penis. He didn't say what it was but drew a child and said he would put it in his mouth. He also drew a can of fizzy drink and said he would be given it by "Hassan", one of the adolescents who had become a cause of concern, later that day. Understandably, Eleni found such a graphic and immediate picture very distressing. Although young children's drawings do not necessarily correlate with actual events and are infused with fantasy, it is highly unusual for such a concrete and explicit drawing like this except in cases of abuse. It was as close as Farid could get to a disclosure and description of what was happening. The disturbing reality it represented was shockingly present. Eleni brought it to supervision and then reported it as a serious concern to management and also to their team meeting. Vigilance was increased at the shelter, including a very demanding 24-hour rota for an already stretched and exhausted staff team.

What was in some senses almost as shocking but driven by the group defence against anxiety described above was what happened over the following week. Doubts were raised at all levels by colleagues and management. "It was a picture only. It didn't mean that anything was happening". "Maybe it just related to what had happened to Farid in the camp". "Perhaps he was confused?" As the doubts set in, so did the undermining of Eleni's confidence. She returned to supervision, saying, "we don't really know what happened". This dynamic was explored with Eleni, including the reality that although there would never be absolute certainty, there was clearly such a high level of risk that the team needed to maintain its vigilance and to keep working on boundaries and norms in the shelter. These conversations became increasingly frank with both staff and children in the shelter, including with Farid. The concern was raised with Hassan, who denied that anything had happened but accepted being moved to another shelter, but this time with older adolescents only. Farid also gradually understood that he could turn to dependable adults for comfort, food, and any "treats" without any sexualised and exploitative transaction. In the remaining couple of months that Eleni and her team worked with Farid, although the concern remained very high and he continued to act out in other ways, they managed to maintain these boundaries and no further incidents with him were reported. Farid also spent a few weeks going to a small local school which had places for asylum-seeking children, where it was noted that he began to play, at times, more normally and appropriately for his age. Pressure had also been placed on the asylum lawyers to try to accelerate Farid's case and he was moved to another charity on the mainland in early 2021. Contact was lost and it is uncertain what happened to him there.

Between "getting one's hands dirty" and "turning a blind eye"

More ordinarily, abuse and exploitation may be thought of as acts between individual perpetrators and victims. However, children like Farid were dependent on dysfunctional systems that were nested in an environment saturated with hostility, abuse, and exploitation, and in which norms had been eroded. In some senses, it could be argued that his story, and his picture, represented not only his own predicament but the context as a whole.

It is, of course, quite clear that this was less than ideal work. The frequent failures to protect, deeply disturbing as they were, could feel as if one was colluding with the abuse and exploitation itself, as described earlier. Organisations and charities working with asylum-seeking children in this context were too overwhelmed, under-resourced and under siege to adequately meet their duty of care. There was no ultimate containing meta-structure or sense of accountability for these children at much higher levels of political responsibility. Arguably, those in positions of power were themselves active in the persecution. In these situations, "horizontal" networks and solidarity groups attempting to protect these children can be formed, but there is no "vertical" line of responsibility that can provide the necessary containment of anxieties or even a sense of secure delegated authority that are a prerequisite for sustained adequate functioning when doing this work.

With little containment, this leaves professionals, like "Ray of Hope's" psychologists, exposed to perpetual oscillations between either extremely persecuted or extremely guilty states of mind, with no sense of a way through, only a way out. The intensity of the work and the emotional exhaustion it caused was, from a psychoanalytic perspective, partly a result of these oscillations between paranoid-schizoid and depressive positions. In an environment such as the one described in this chapter, the former (paranoid-schizoid states of mind) meant intense fears of being persecuted or attacked, accused, and condemned for something unforgivable and suffering reputational damage or destruction as a result. Individuals, and the organisations they worked in, felt unprotected from these terrors and from the risk of being scapegoated. The broader systemic failure to protect these children's basic human rights was at times projected into them. In short, the very people who were trying to do something were blamed.

Intensely persecuted states of mind lead to splitting, denial, and projection – emotionally cutting off, blaming others, and walking away – or "turning a blind eye". If such pressures and anxiety could be withstood, with support, then there arose the possibility of moving towards "depressive anxieties", remaining concerned and engaged, but which also meant at times the awful burden of intense guilt about the situation – a feeling that one was "getting one's hands dirty" by staying involved. This is the central dilemma that I believe these teams faced. Get involved but then feel complicit in an abusive, corrupt, and exploitative system; or turn a blind eye and walk away. From a Kleinian perspective, the former, though fragile and "contaminated", is the more psychologically mature and ethically developed position. It means a great deal of hard psychological work to face one's split core and avow what has been disavowed, including one's own destructiveness. At the same time, it means experiencing repetitive depressive anxieties – the repeated loss of a sense of hope and goodness, including one's own – a long and painful disillusionment, which risks being traumatic in itself (Steiner, 2018). Though disavowal may thus look like the easier course, what is lost is one's "integrity", in the fullest sense of the term, through this splitting and fragmentation of consciousness or awareness. We lose the capacity to bear, and, therefore, work through guilt and shame and forfeit the possibility of engaging with the sometimes-terrible knowledge that they indicate.

Supervision potentially offered a space that could run counter to the turning of a blind eye, at least temporarily, but this meant opening up psychic pain – shame and guilt; putting "Ray of Hope's" psychologists, back in touch with an awareness of destructive forces and the damage these forces were causing – in the environment and systems they were working in, in the young people they were working with, and in themselves. This also meant getting in contact with potentially traumatising experiences that were being defended against; the risk of feeling flooded, overwhelmed, and psychically attacked; experiences of helplessness, terror, rage, and despair.

If these could be contained, supervision could provide further space for the working through of depressive anxieties, which was necessary for the mobilisation of reparative impulses and a sense of responsibility for the damaged psychic space that was apparent. This meant that whilst this endured, it helped to provide a safeguard against the slippage of various norms and the protection they provided. These included countering the pervasive denial of these children's dependency and the general erosion of an ordinary understanding of developmental needs and developmental trauma; working against the deterioration in expectations that were beginning to allow the expression of various forms of hostility towards the children, including racialised exchanges and intimidation; and reinforcing the prohibitions against psychically destructive sexual behaviour and sexual transgressions.

These efforts were subject to repeated failure. However, this is not to say that they were not of some value, even if they offered only limited and temporary protection for children like Farid. This is unsurprising in the broader context described in this chapter. Supervision also bears witness to what happens and provides some recognition for the intense emotional work done in these environments. In a small way, this chapter bears witness to the collective violence towards, and abuse and exploitation of, unaccompanied asylum-seeking children in general, and seeks to recognise the exhausting and courageous work of professionals like "Ray of Hope's" psychology teams.

Notes

1 Here, the meaning of "good parents" is not restricted to biological parents but can refer to any majorly significant attachment figures involved in the care, protection, nurture, and upbringing of the child.
2 According to Jones (2017, p. 16), more than half the deaths at borders globally, in the decade to 2015, occurred at the edges of the EU.
3 For example, see the UNHCR and Save the Children UK assessment of the sexual violence and exploitation of refugee children in West Africa under UN protection: "The agencies that are possibly implicated in some way include UN peacekeeping forces, international and local NGOs, and government agencies responsible for humanitarian response" (UNHCR, 2002, p. 2).

References

Amnesty International (2021). *"Greece: Violence, lies, and pushbacks – Refugees and migrants still denied safety and asylum at Europe's borders"*. Amnesty International.

Ayotte, W. (2000). *Separated Children Coming to Western Europe: Why They Travel and How They Arrive (vol. 3)*. London: Save the Children.

Barn, R., Di Rosa, T. and Kallinikaki, T. (2021). *Unaccompanied minors in Greece and Italy: An exploration of the challenges for social work within tighter immigration and resource constraints in pandemic times*. Social Sciences, 10, 134. https://doi.org/10.3390/socsci10040134

Berry, M., Garcia-Blanco, I., Moore, K., Morani, M., Gross, B., Askanius, T. and Linné, T. (2015). *Press coverage of the refugee and migrant crisis in the EU: A content analysis of five European countries*. Cardiff School of Journalism. http://www.unhcr.org/56bb369c9.html

Bhabha, J. (2014). *Child Migration and Human Rights in a Global Age*. Princeton, NJ: Princeton University Press.

Chase, E. (2020). *Transitions, capabilities, and wellbeing: How Afghan unaccompanied young people experience becoming "adult" in the UK and beyond*. Journal of Ethnic and Migration Studies, 46, 439–456.

Digidiki, V. and Bhabha, J. (2018). *Sexual abuse and exploitation of unaccompanied migrant children in Greece: Identifying risk factors and gaps in services during the European migration crisis.* Children and Youth Services Review, Elsevier, 92: 114–121.

Freccero, J., Biswas, D., Whiting, A., Alrabe, K. and Seelinger, K.T. (2017). *Sexual exploitation of unaccompanied migrant and refugee boys in Greece: Approaches to prevention.* PLoS Med, 14 (11): e1002438. https://doi.org/10.1371/journal.pmed.1002438

House of Lords (2016). *Children in crisis: Unaccompanied migrant children in the EU.* https://publications.parliament.uk/pa/ld201617/ldselect/ldeucom/34/34.pdf

IFRC (International Federation of Red Cross and Red Crescent Societies) (2018). *Alone and unsafe. Children, migration, and sexual and gender-based violence.* Document released online 05.12.2018. https://www.ifrc.org/sites/default/files/181126-AloneUnsafe-Report-EN-web.pdf

IRC (International Rescue Committee) (2020). Cruelty of containment | International Rescue Committee (IRC). https://www.rescue.org/sites/default/files/2020-12/IRC_Cruelty_of_Containment_FINAL.pdf

Jones, R. (2017). *Violent Borders: Refugees and the Right to Move.* London: Verso.

Medicins Sans Frontières (2022). Greece | Our Work & How to Help | Doctors Without Borders – USA.

Papadopoulos, R. (2002). *Therapeutic Care for Refugees: No Place Like Home.* Oxford: Routledge.

Steiner, J. (1985). *Turning a blind eye: The cover up for Oedipus.* International Review of Psychoanalysis, 12, 161–172.

Steiner, J. (2018). *The trauma and disillusionment of Oedipus.* The International Journal of Psychoanalysis, 99:3, 555–568.

Sto Nisi (2020). «Επιβεβαίωση της αναγκαιότητας δημιουργίας κλειστών και ελεγχόμενων δομών» | StoNisi.gr

UNCRC (1989). *United Nations Convention on the rights of the child.* https://www.unicef.org.uk/wp-content/uploads/2016/08/unicef-convention-rights-child-uncrc.pdf

UNHCR (2002). Note for Implementing and Operational Partners by UNHCR and Save the Children-UK on Sexual Violence & Exploitation: The Experience of Refugee Children in Guinea, Liberia, and Sierra Leone | UNHCR.

12

COMMUNITY PSYCHOTHERAPY

Creating a therapeutic culture in frontline care organisations

Ariel Nathanson

In his paper "the antisocial tendency", Winnicott (1968) describes how a highly destructive patient was violent to him and even stole his car. Winnicott uses this patient as an example of a very deprived child who needed "management" rather than psychotherapy. He suggests that young people who are highly antisocial and destructive in their behaviour cannot be successfully treated in psychotherapy. More importantly, psychotherapy is not enough to tackle the deprivation at the core of their antisocial behaviour. Change can only be achieved through transforming their environment so their needs can be noticed and addressed by the people who look after them.

The patients I usually work with in psychotherapy or hear about as a consultant are similar to the type of patient described by Winnicott. In fact, these patients have come to represent a much larger section of referrals, requiring networks of professionals to manage and look after them. These disturbed young people hardly ever receive long-term psychological treatment and indeed, as Winnicott suggested, are unlikely to engage or benefit from it. In addition, many of them are never noticed by anyone outside their immediate environment. Without an opportunity to feel safe and create new positive attachments, their pathological solutions developed in the context of their relational trauma become the structure at the core of their evolving personalities.

As Winnicott suggests, deprived young people disturb others as a way of calling attention to their unmet needs. However, their calls are often not heard or heard by the wrong people and organisations. As a generalisation, therefore, perpetrators are likely to elicit punitive responses from statutory services that would attempt to protect others from them or be taken in by those who would offer them protection in exchange for loyalty to a destructive criminal aim. Victims, on the other hand, elicit a wish to save and protect

DOI: 10.4324/9781003020370-12

but collude with their perpetrators, attempting to master their abuse and deprivation by further victimisation and self-destructiveness.

As anyone working in the field of mental health and care knows, relational trauma is often intergenerational. As such, it impacts the lives of many people, even whole communities. Deprivation, addiction, criminality, and physical illness are highly associated with each other. Some experts and activists even advocate addressing them as a public health issue, which indeed makes much sense. It is obvious that attempting to solve these issues by addressing individual problems while neglecting the environment is unlikely to make a real difference. Staying loyal to Winnicott's general ideas, only by either changing the environment or providing a totally new one can real change be experienced.

Frontline care workers might have the capacity to provide some of this help and work within this ethos. They are usually found close to those who need help, at times even before they are able to ask for it. Yet, these workers are often offered very little support to carry out a complicated and disturbing task. As a result, similar to the young people who had to develop pathological solutions to survive their trauma, frontline care workers hold on to organisational defences (Menzies-Lyth, 1988) that separate them from the trauma associated with their relational work, rendering their interventions too contrived and therefore ineffective.

In this chapter, I would like to offer a model of consultation and training focused on creating and enhancing the therapeutic aspects of the relationships frontline professionals make with traumatised and severely disturbed young people. In my experience, employing this model successfully narrows the gap between disturbed young people and the therapy they need by providing it on the front line by those already there. As I write this chapter, I imagine the readers to be the frontline professionals I usually consult to, their managers, social workers, educators, and policymakers. In parallel, I also write to psychotherapists like me who are interested in developing expertise in providing this type of consultative work.

As this book focuses on exploitation, I have chosen my illustrations to represent this experience. Although this is not the theme of this chapter, I thought that it might help connect it to the rest of the book and shed some light on how the consultation model of work can contribute to an environmental approach to helping victims of exploitation and many others.

I will start by describing a typical scene in a therapeutic consultation in order to give a first glance into how this looks and what it feels like. I will adopt several points of view, as in the consultation itself, following the way it usually unfolds, looking for projections and fragmented experiences within the practices of individual members of staff, their group, their leaders, and the organisational dynamic.

Donna, a sixteen-year-old adolescent girl, has recently moved out from her foster placement to semi-independent supported accommodation following a placement breakdown. In the year leading to the breakdown, Donna started absconding for long periods of time, and it was suspected that she had been meeting men that she linked with on various online platforms. There was also some suspicion that she was being paid for sex because she seemed to have some money in her possession, which she used to buy fashionable clothes and trainers. As she was only fifteen at the time, the police became involved, but Donna did not cooperate with the investigation and refused to divulge what she had been doing or whom she had been doing it with.

Her foster parents of three years, to whom she was attached, were unable to tolerate her growing contempt of them as well as not being able to protect her from the risk she was putting herself in. She was described as "hyper and out of control".

As in many other cases, Donna suffered a history of abuse and neglect. Her mother was seventeen at the time of her birth and spent a year in supportive foster care with her baby, where she was reported to be doing well. However, when the young mother moved out, she got back together with Donna's father, who was a member of a known gang. He was violent to Donna's mother for a couple of years before being sent to prison for a long period. During this time, their little council flat became a gang-den, with strangers visiting to buy and consume drugs. It was always suspected but never proven that Donna was not only neglected by her mother, who was now herself victimised and colluding with the gang, but also sexually abused herself. Obviously, in that environment of drugs and violence, there was no benign adult to keep baby Donna safe and cared for.

Donna moved into foster care aged five, but by the age of ten, her first placement broke down following the death of her foster father. She settled well in her second placement but started to deteriorate after transferring to secondary school. Aged thirteen, a video of her giving oral sex to a group of boys in the school was circulated. After a period off school, feeling ashamed and enraged, Donna returned to school with an older adolescent boy who violently attacked one of the boys in the video. Donna was expelled and moved to a local Pupil Referral Unit. A sharp escalation in her behaviour that culminated in the second placement breaking down started at that point.

Her third placement was a well-staffed semi-independent accommodation, part of a larger organisation providing residential care and a fostering agency. This was the context of the consultation where Donna's case was discussed.

Donna's female link-worker felt that she had made good contact with her. However, the link-worker was a bit dismissive, describing Donna as enjoying a risky lifestyle and experimenting with various relationships, denying the risk Donna was in. Two male members of staff acknowledged that Donna was over-sexualised and had directly tried to seduce them. They had reacted by trying to avoid her in fear of allegations. Another female member of staff, somewhat overweight, felt very hurt by Donna, who always referred to her as "the meat". This was news to the staff group, who reacted with surprise that this had never been discussed before. The staff member concerned responded by saying she thought that she could deal with it herself but then admitted that she was contemplating leaving the organisation.

In consultation, I made sure that the staff group was able to discuss the history of the case. Sharing the details of abuse and trauma is often very shocking but essential to creating a narrative that provides better understanding of the current presentation. The professional group developed a vivid image of baby Donna in the violent drug-den, frightened and unprotected. It was then possible to start thinking about how she tried to protect herself from pain – by psychologically joining those who not only turned a blind eye to her abuse but also denigrated her infantile needs. The group was able to transpose the picture of Donna's infancy onto the current enactments and see the adolescent as the omnipotent baby in control of the gang-den, mastering her abuse by becoming seductive and then quickly using the money she got to buy the "bling" she covered herself with, both as an armour, and as if inhabiting a gangster from within.

Through the consultation, the various fragments of Donna's projections could be recognised as lodged within different members of staff; her linkworker held on to a dismissive Donna who turned a blind eye to the risk she was in, in order to avoid feeling unprotected and vulnerable. The male care workers experienced Donna's attempt at mastering her trauma by being seductive and by initiating the sexual contact over which she had once had no control. The victimised member of staff was the worst affected, as she held the most painful aspects of the trauma; she felt the impact of the cruel Donna who was in identification with the abusive gang, and the victim Donna's vulnerability, isolation, and inability to ask for help, and her difficulty in accessing benign and protective aggression. As these fragments were collected and deciphered, they made a full picture, fitting both the infantile trauma and the current enactments. It was also noticeable how staff members' experiences were shaped not only by Donna's projections but also by their own internal lives and relational histories. It was as though Donna scattered her projections, and they each picked up the ones that fitted them best – the projections they could not process but had matched experiences of their own which they were used to tolerating and coping with.

With the personal and group dynamics now attended to, the raw ingredients of the original trauma were laid bare. The staff were now disturbed but less traumatised and entangled in Donna's rigid defence system. They had something to contain rather than just be activated by and could use their group and leaders as a container for their own disturbance.

At the core of the consultation model is the idea of containment as described by Bion (1962). Containment is a very active state of mind. As Bion suggested, it is the main developmental ingredient in the mother–infant relationship. The mother relates to her infant's extreme states of mind, absorbs them, feels disturbed by them, and then thinks and acts in order to meet her infant's needs. It is the most ordinary of human experiences and emotional life, yet a radical act of love that enables the development of an ability to tolerate emotional experiences and think before taking action. As most of the young people we hear about and work with do the opposite – cannot tolerate emotional states, do not reflect, and act impulsively without thinking – containment is obviously at the core of what they missed out on, and is what they need the most.

Getting to know a very disturbed or anxious mind is a shock to one's relational system and structure. Ordinarily, we expect people to be able to tell us what's wrong and how they feel. If they are very young, we expect them to show distress and be available to receive comfort. We do not tend to imagine a reality in which intense distress, dread, and other difficult states of mind are violently projected, overwhelming our own internal containers, inducing emotions and experiences that might even challenge the way we perceive ourselves.

I believe that becoming available to experience and contain these projections is a radical act similar to the transition adults go through when they become parents. From being primarily psychological projectors who expect to be contained, they are suddenly overwhelmed by an infant's radical projections of raw infantile needs, which they need to contain. The result is usually a dramatic stretching of an internal container, now fit to hold on to extreme states of mind, hopefully without evoking unhelpful unconscious dramas of the past.

Those starting to work in residential care, for example, often describe a similar shock when they suddenly experience the gap between their fantasies about the work and the actual experience. Care staff who have learned about attachment and might have experienced security in their own psychological development are tasked with looking after those who needed to survive chronic rejection, fear, and abuse. Indeed, having been looked after well enables one to develop a way of containing others adequately. However, it does not prepare workers for being attacked and denigrated and for living in fear. In addition, those who might have suffered their own childhood traumas and difficulties are suddenly and very powerfully thrown back into states of psychological emergency and find themselves resorting to their own pathological defences and enactments.

Feeling disturbed by these radical experiences is part of the role and experience of being in contact with severely traumatised young people. Obviously, disturbance is necessary for containment to occur, and containment is what fuels emotional and psychological development and recovery.

Organisational therapeutic consultation

The therapeutic consultation model I offer, first developed by Jenny Sprince (2002), is focused on enhancing the capacity to contain by paying very close attention to all aspects of an organisation's relational life. Those depend on three main strands: (1) the histories, traumas, and their expression in the people the organisation is tasked to look after or treat; (2) the histories, traumas, and personalities of individual staff members and the way this comes across in relationships to young people and colleagues; and (3) the group and organisational dynamics, organisational culture and task, individual professional identities, trainings, and responsibilities.

The radical changes in containing capacity needed for therapeutically looking after very disturbed young people require special organisational arrangements. As described by Sprince, this type of containment should be provided in rings circling each other; in the focus is the young person (and/or group of young people). Around them, providing the first contact is the individual worker on the front line. Around him or her are the immediate staff group, the small team, and its leader. Surrounding them is a wider staff group led by more experienced leaders with more authority. Around all of these is the organisation, structuring these relationships and providing the setting where containment can be available. Obviously, a structure is not enough. The individuals, groups, and their relationships to each other are what make the real environment – the people using the structure. This can be very nurturing when it functions well and quite toxic when it does not.

Case example

I would like to describe another case in some more detail in order to show how the model works and especially how the therapeutic organisational consultant addresses all levels of the organisation from the individual resident, the staff member, and then the group and the organisation as a whole.

This is a composite of many different young people I have heard about over the years. The context is a residential care home attempting to create a therapeutic environment.

Young people are usually placed in residential care only as a last resort after repeated failures of foster care placements. As a result, they are not only suffering the impact of infantile relational trauma but are also veterans of many subsequent failures, at times presenting as highly omnipotent masters of placement destruction, needing containment but acting to destroy anyone attempting to offer it to them.

The consultant learns who the young people are through the eyes and experiences of the care workers, never by working with them or assessing them directly. It is made clear from the very beginning that the consultant is not there to treat the young people or assess them, or dictate the way they should be worked with. This boundary should never be crossed. It is essential in order to preserve the focus on the staff's experience and on the organisational dynamic. Additionally, it allows the staff to further develop their authority as the ones who know the young people best, can represent their needs and work therapeutically with them.

One of the principles of the consultation is to challenge the split between what is considered care and what is seen as therapy and to develop a new role and task – therapeutic care. In order to foster the creation of such a culture, the consultation has to adhere to a structure and boundaries that facilitate it. For example, the consultant cannot offer direct work to the young people in order to avoid a culture in which the consultant becomes the expert, and the care staff is there to follow prescriptions. As in psychotherapy, the consultant's role is not to tell people what to do but to help staff develop their own therapeutic authority and thinking. It also supports the general idea that young people suffering high levels of trauma and disturbance can only be treated in a total therapeutic environment, receiving around the clock therapy in every aspect of their lives rather than a weekly therapy session surrounded by daily care.

Connor

Thirteen-year-old Connor became seductive when approached by residential care staff. While they felt that they were offering physical comfort to a distressed boy, he interpreted their closeness as a threat and pre-empted this by attempting to sexualise the contact. Closeness evoked his trauma and confusion. His solution was to master it through taking a masochistic position that invited pain, rather than anxiously waiting for it. When he realised that he could not sexualise his relationship with staff members, his anxiety escalated rather than diminished: he felt on uncharted, unpredictable territory where adults behaved in ways he could not master and control. As a result, as is the case for many other similar children, he felt driven to escalate his behaviour so as to feel in control again. When he became violent, he evoked a predictable reaction from the adults; he needed to be physically restrained. But the staff reported that they noticed that while they were having to hold him, he became sexually excited. His excitement led him to escalate the situation still further, and workers reported feeling scared of him. Some then felt compelled to placate him in order to preserve a quiet shift. Others became quite punitive, secretly, or unconsciously using physical restraint as a punishment, a way of "getting back control" rather than as a means of restoring safety. It became very clear that one shift's calm was another shift's catastrophe and that the team needed to make better sense of the overall dynamic. Some members of staff seemed to feel victimised themselves, first by the young person and then by the organisation and their managers who, according to them, failed to protect them from Connor. They acted out by making mistakes such as forgetting the car keys in the kitchen, not locking away matches, knives, and even medication. Unable to regulate, Connor felt compelled to act when he noticed these objects. It was as though the staff had given Connor the means by which he could both victimise them and hurt himself.

A very central dynamic to this work, as described by Docker-Drysdale (1968), is indeed the oscillation or splitting in the staff group between becoming highly punitive, demanding harsh consequences to bad behaviour, and acting in a placatory way, seeing only the victim, and attempting to pacify the perpetrator, usually in order to "preserve the peace". Similar oscillations in the countertransference will also be familiar to psychotherapists working individually with violent patients.

Finding a third way that is neither of those extreme enactments is a therapeutic task that creates the potential for developing a better way of relating. It is, in fact, one of the main aims of the consultation and of the culture it creates and supports.

Integrating experiences: The young person – individual staff member – group – organisation

A consultation day often seems to follow a theme, which might emerge at some point or in hindsight. It is seldom linear, but for the purpose of this chapter, I would like to relate such a theme separately to the individual staff member, then the group, and eventually the organisational dynamic.

I have already described Connor's disturbance and how it directly impacted the staff and challenged their capacities to understand, contain, and react to him.

I would now like to start with discussing the way looking after this boy impacted on an individual member of staff and show how the consultation addresses personal difficulties in the context of the work. I will then turn to the group and finally to the organisation.

The individual member of staff

One staff member looking after Connor found it difficult to sleep before a shift and even had panic attacks prior to driving to work in the morning. Her practice was avoidant. She kept her distance from the boy and was placatory when she sensed that a conflict might be brewing. In many ways, she presented with symptoms associated with PTSD or what is now termed "compassion fatigue" (Figley, 2002).

In an individual consultation session, which she requested, the staff member spoke about her own history of growing up scared of her father, who used to be extremely strict and violent to her mother and brothers, though never to her. She was then helped to see how her old solutions to managing her own experience – avoiding, hiding, and pacifying – were no longer viable in the context of her role and made her feel stuck. She did not feel that she had any other way of dealing with violence, so she became terrified of the boy, now embodying her father, and panicked.

Following the consultation, where she felt contained, she was able to talk to her team leader and later her group. Others spoke about different personal experiences, and all shared the idea that they, too, had individual ways of coping with violence, which shaped the manner they related to the young person they were caring for.

Significantly, this way of consulting or supervising someone's professional work might be quite alien to psychotherapists, as in the consultation, there is no clear split between the personal, which psychotherapists are expected to take to their psychoanalysis, and the professional, expected to be explored in supervision.

The consultation purposefully combines individual and professional development by welcoming discussions and disclosures from staff about their personal experiences in the context of their roles. In doing so it provides what Jenny Sprince (https://psychodynamicthinking.info/appcios-therapeutic-supervision) calls *therapeutic supervision*; the opportunity to reflect on one's own experiences as they are provoked and emerge through the work. The consultant attends to projections originating from the young person while in parallel analysing the staff member's specific valency[1] to being disturbed and unconsciously activated by them.

In fact, if we cared to look, we might find that any staff group is populated by ghosts (Fraiberg, Adelson and Shapiro, 1975) of the staff's past interacting with those of the young people in their care and impacting on their relationships to each other. Although the organisational task is to address the ghosts populating the minds of disturbed young people, it is the consultation's task to enable this by not neglecting all the other ghosts and unconscious processes.

Individual experiences do not only emerge in reaction to difficult young people. They are often linked to relationships in the team and especially with authority figures, naturally evoking unconscious dramas and responses. With time, the consultant gets to know the staff in a very personal way, with some akin to therapy, at least in periods of personal transition and change. This integral part of the consultation can become quite therapeutic for the people engaged in it as they turn corners in their relationships to their roles, to the young people, to the organisation, and to themselves.

The group

The individual staff member described earlier took an active part in splitting the team; she and a few others felt victimised by Connor and campaigned for more protection from the organisation, urging the organisation to discharge him as too dangerous. Others agreed but felt that Connor was "getting away with too much" and advocated more behavioural consequences. Although feeling quite alienated from the manager, the care staff breathed a collective sigh of relief when she was around and was herself relating to Connor directly.

They called upon her to intervene, which she did, making them feel temporarily protected. They hated her when she went home in the evening and were extremely resentful when she came back, unconsciously showing her their devastation at being left with Connor overnight or during a weekend.

In their team consultation, the staff were helped to see how their wish for a quiet shift mirrored the boy's experience and fear, his need to placate in order to survive, along with his feelings of resentment and his inability to use aggression in a protective way. Others understood how overpoweringly Connor represented their inability to tolerate humiliation. As the staff group was able to contain its individual members who presented as more sensitive and fearful of Connor's violence, they became better professionals; firm without being punitive and understanding without being placatory.

The organisation

The manager and the leadership team were keen to hold on to Connor and used their experience and authority to attend to him when they were around. Indeed, as long as the manager was in the home the boy did not behave in an "unmanageable" way. However, when the manager left at five, Connor became more challenging, and then the evening shift would either ring the manager at home or call the police. When the manager arrived in the morning, she would find the home in a mess and feel that she needed to micro-manage the staff rather than rely on the shift leaders. She began to see them as weak ("it was never like this in my time") and felt quite punitive, translating her own way of dealing with Connor into step-by-step procedures she wanted the staff to follow, especially when she was not there.

In an individual session with the manager at the end of the consultation day, she was helped to see how over-involved she had become in the life of the young people in the home and in micro-managing the staff. She felt torn between feeling she had to protect her staff, worried that they might leave, and angry that they did not seem to take on their responsibilities and needed her too much. She felt misunderstood and victimised by the staff and persecuted by a highly critical social worker (who herself felt persecuted by her own department). She was tempted to bully her staff into action by creating a very tight structure to abide by in the same way that she felt bullied to "protect" them by the combined invisible threat that they would leave, and that the social worker would remove the boy. It was possible to show a thread connecting the boy's unconscious experiences with that of the staff group and the organisation, all impacting on the manager. As a result of the consultation session, she felt encouraged to liaise more frequently with the leadership team and share the burden rather than try to protect them. In a wider discussion with the team, the issue of people threatening to leave was raised and discussed. The manager spoke about how they needed to take up more authority themselves rather than relying only on hers. Now freer to act within their roles, rather than at the mercy of individual and group unconscious dynamics, the staff were ready to be led and to face the young person from a position of containing and firm authority.

Organisational defences

Menzies-Lyth (1988) described the ways in which a hospital ward "protected" the nurses by providing various organisational structures and practices that when followed reduced or eliminated the nurses' anxiety relating to their work with ill children, some of whom would not survive their illnesses. Menzies-Lyth also showed how the organisation substituted the original anxieties stemming from the nurses' relationships with the ill children with what she termed *secondary anxieties* and defined as "threats of crisis and operational breakdown", which preoccupied the nurses and management, instead of the relational anxiety linked to the work itself.

Keeping in mind the dynamic I described in the organisation I consulted to, it is easy to see how without the consultation the organisation could have become very defensive. The manager would have continued to cement her expectations from the staff into further formal controlling procedures, which in turn would have provided the staff with a distraction from the relational focus of their work. They might that have felt persecuted about fulfilling their procedural duties and have spent less time with Connor rather than feeling frightened by the relational impact of the work. In time, as the structure matured, it would have gained rigidity, functioning as a barrier between the staff and the young people and mediating their contact so that challenges and relational conflicts would have been reduced. In parallel, the manager's anxieties about children being removed and about the overall reputation of the organisation would have been channelled directly into the staff, who would have started to worry about the survival of the organisation and the future of their employment. These two types of defences would then have been likely to complement each other; the anxiety about relating to the young people, surviving their attacks, and containing their projections would have been transformed into a concern about the organisation's survival. Slowly but surely, the organisational task of looking after and treating severely traumatised young people would have been covertly transformed into the task of preserving the survival of the organisation itself. The children's needs would have been subordinated to the needs of the organisation, and the task of looking after them would have been harnessed as an instrument in the organisation's fight for existence.

If the consultation process works well and continues to be supported, over time, the relational way of containing anxiety becomes the organisational culture, rendering organisational defences no longer desperately needed. This does not mean that workers will be left to the mercy of violent young people without protection or exposed to social workers and auditors who see them as ineffective. It means that they will feel supported in fully engaging with young people by developing their own authority and courage based on a growing capacity to contain primitive states of mind.

Community psychotherapy – the development of relational thinking and practice on the frontline

I recently asked a youth worker what she thought her role was as part of a professional network meeting to discuss a young person she worked with. Her reply, after an initial coy "I don't know", was to say that she always felt the "odd one out", almost as if she were another troubled young person rather than part of the professional network. However, as our discussion developed and she felt freer to think and evaluate what she knew about the young person in question, it became very clear that she held both the most information and the best relationship. She was the only member of the professional network that the young person trusted.

Part of this worker's difficulty in feeling professional was the relationship she had with her own role. When asked if her work was therapeutic, she hesitated, said no, and then, in a small child voice added "maybe?". As this was part of a consultation to the service she worked for, some of her colleagues identified with her experiences and contributed their own. It was noticeable that they never felt professional and thought that this was part of what enabled them to make good relationships with young people and be trusted by them. In fact, quite a few of them said that they were not too sure whether they belonged to the adult world just yet and felt more at ease with the young people they worked with than with the teachers, social workers, and counsellors they met as part of their formal role. Although they described this as a strength, which indeed it was, they also agreed that if they could feel more at ease in the adult professional world then they could become intermediaries, representing the young people they cared for to the professionals rather than identify with the young people and feel infantilised, not-heard, resentful and angry.

As described earlier in this chapter, the consultation model to residential care creates and maintains a relational organisational culture. With time, this culture no longer depends on the consultant and its association with him or her. It is an integral part of the structure and identity of anyone working in the organisation. As Jenny Sprince (2002) noticed, the consultation is both a therapeutic endeavour and a professional training. As the organisation begins to heal so do individual members of staff, all benefitting from exploring their personal relationships to their roles, the young people, and the institutional dynamic. As they do so over a few years, they develop a new professional identity, that of an Organisational Psychotherapist, delivering therapeutic support to people within an organisational setting.

Psychoanalytic consultation provided to frontline workers of any denomination, both the skilled and formally educated and the unskilled graduates of their own experiences, can expand the culture of therapeutic thinking. As the consultation develops and the organisation becomes more containing and less defensive, some space can be created in which the consultation can evolve into a more structured training.

The training itself, like the consultation, can be tailor made. Its focus must remain the consultation in the context of the actual work and organisational task. However, a few more modules of learning can be added, some provided by the consultant and some by others who can run specific seminars. Main topics to be added might include a reading theory seminar and an observation seminar (usually infant, young child, and/or organisational observation).

Those who have attended the consultation for a while enjoy the opportunity to start conceptualising their experiential learning so far. It gives them a language to start communicating their understanding and formulate their thinking to others.

Indeed, many organisations describe themselves as "therapeutic" and "trauma and attachment focused". Their staff attend trainings in trauma and attachment and neuroscience, learning and developing their understanding in those topics. However, as I have noticed many times, although the trainings and trainers are very good, the learning remains disconnected from the actual experience of working on the front line.

I do not think that it is possible to offer people sporadic training in thinking and working in a relational way, attachment–focused, trauma–aware, and expect that this will impact practice right away. Those attending these trainings may enjoy them and learn a bit more but are likely to continue working in exactly the same way.

The only way to make a real impact and effect change is to offer containment (Bion, 1962) through intensive, long-term personal and organisational consultation. Only then, especially once the consultation evolves into training, are the staff able to talk about their work as therapeutic and explain why it is. Those who choose to take this forward can become registered as organisational therapists, a professional identity already accepted and recognised by the British Psychoanalytic Council.

In residential care, those holding this title and experience can become better leaders and supervisors of other staff. They now represent an organisational therapeutic culture and practice embodied in their roles. The leadership and containment they can offer their staff and the traumatised young people they work with are invaluable and long lasting.

The consultation-as-a-course can also be provided outside a coherent organisation that has employed a consultant. In order to recreate the consultation experience, the course can be structures to resemble a long-term group relations event. As members of the learning group start to participate and to share their experiences, they notice the links between their professional experiences outside the group, the relationships they create within the group, and the learning provided within theory seminars. To supplement their experience, they can be provided with therapeutic supervision, additional theory seminars, and observation seminars. With time, many members of such groups seek further psychotherapy as they notice more about themselves and decide to take a closer look.

My experience of providing such courses outside the clear framework of consultation has been interesting and mixed. One group of youth workers mostly working with violent young people developed in a very personal way; members of the group, who were quite traumatised themselves and came from very similar backgrounds to those of their clients, used the course therapeutically. As a result, quite a few of them moved out of their roles to take on a life away from intense contact with trauma and abuse. Others chose to become more professional and opt for extra training in known training institutions. Only a minority retained their original roles, but these members grew in personal authority, and moved to more senior positions in the organisations they came from.

Another training group of people mostly working within education, has been better able to create the group experiential–educational culture in a way that kept them together, maybe because the members of this group came from less traumatised backgrounds. Although this group is currently ongoing, it is already clear that the model is transferable and can be tailor-made to suit the needs of many different frontline workers.

Imagining that therapeutic training can be provided on the front line by combining experiential, professional, and educational experiences might be surprising for experienced psychotherapists reading this chapter. Indeed, our experience is very different; we choose to train, usually start with going to psychoanalysis and then join a training institution representing a specific school of thought. Our psychoanalysis usually lasts for many years, often after our training ends. We are usually part of training groups of people very similar to us in education at least, but often in skin colour and class. Almost all the psychotherapists I have met are liberals belonging to the political left. Only a tiny minority is religious, for example.

Consulting and providing this training on the front line is very different. As a consultant, I am often the odd one out, not fitting into the environment I am in. As an example, I have already been (to name a few) the only Jew in the group, the only white person and the only secular person in a group of devoted believers. Yet the internalisation of containment as an experience and as a concept is no different. The experience of working with trauma is no different, and indeed, there is no difference to the experience of thinking psychoanalytically.

Being consulted to and becoming a member of a consultation-training group is very personal as much as it is professional. People change within their identities and usually become intermediaries, bridging gaps between cultures and experiences rather than being only on one side of the divide.

Therapy, too, does not need to be the privilege of the lucky few. Indeed, as Sprince (2002) observed during her consultative work and as I have seen in mine, individual therapy is often not advisable for young people in residential care. Many others, in communities, prisons, schools, and other settings, might never be able to make the journey (geographical and psychological) needed to access services. However, although long-term psychotherapy has become very rare, therapy within other long-term professional relationships can be developed and enhanced. It can be provided by locally organised frontline workers who receive regular consultation and are using it to develop their psychotherapeutic thinking and to learn from experience.

Note

1 Specific valency is a concept borrowed from chemistry describing the ease with which one element can chemically connect to others. Relationally, it can be described as a personal hook to which projections can attach or what people usually mean when they say that someone is "pressing their buttons".

References

Bion, W.R. (1962). *Learning From Experience*. London, Heinemann.

Docker-Drysdale, B. (1968). *Therapy in Childcare. Collected Papers by Barbara Dockar-Drysdale*. London, Longmans, Green & Co.

Figley, C. (ed) (2002). *Treating Compassion Fatigue*. New York, Brunner-Routledge.

Fraiberg, S., Adelson, E., and Shapiro, V. (1975). *Ghosts in the nursery. A psychoanalytic approach to the problems of impaired infant-mother relationships*. Journal of the American Academy of Child & Adolescent Psychiatry, 14(3), 387–421.

Menzies-Lyth, I. (1988). *Containing Anxiety in Institutions, Vol. 1*. London, Free Association Books.

Sprince, J. (2002). *Developing Containment: Psychoanalytic Consultancy to a Therapeutic Community for Traumatized Children*. Journal of Child Psychotherapy, Vol. 28(2).

Winnicott, D. (1968). *Playing: Its theoretical status in the clinical situation*. The International Journal of Psychoanalysis, 49(4), 591–599.

13

DON'T WE ALL ENVY MOTHERS

Marion Bower

The earlier chapters in this book have described how difficult it is for young people to give up sexually exploitative relationships and how these can have an addictive quality. In this chapter, I explore how very early experiences of emotional deprivation can contribute to vulnerability to exploitation.

There are many causes of early emotional neglect – parental mental illness, drug and alcohol abuse and marital violence are some causes. I use the example of children's experiences of daycare for very explicit demonstrations of how lack of staff attentiveness can create distress and increase children's vulnerability – there is increasing pressure on mothers to take up daycare and return rapidly to work after a new child is born. Paradoxically, children's unhappiness in daycare also affects staff and there can be rapid staff turnover.

Daycare could be simply improved and provide a radically better experience for both tiny children being cared for, and for staff. The random indiscriminate care model is often used in the care system too. The alternative of an identified single adult who acts consistently as a substitute parent for a small group of three or four children can provide an immediate and huge improvement.

'Don't we all envy mothers'. These words were spoken by an intelligent social worker who was due to start an unusual postgraduate course. This was a partnership between a well-regarded postgraduate social work training with a sociological ethos and a specialist psychotherapeutic NHS[1] clinic that was particularly known for its psychoanalytic approach. Political and sociological approaches have generally been located in different institutions from psychoanalytic approaches. Current developments in society have made it helpful for the psychoanalytic and sociological frameworks to speak to each other. An example is the development of gangs of sexual exploiters.

DOI: 10.4324/9781003020370-13

Random daycare

At the time of writing (2023), a conservative government was putting pressure on mothers to put their young children in daycare and return to work. To sweeten this, they promised a 'graduate' in every class. Many nurseries take babies from three months old upwards. A graduate, unless they had relevant qualifications, would have little or nothing to add to the care of babies and very young children except perhaps a delusion that day nurseries could provide education (rather than care) for babies. Research by McGuire and Earls (1994) came to a bleak conclusion about day nurseries. 'Rather than children becoming socialised in nurseries, the opposite is taking place .... The nursery was shown to be the cause of increased aggression and retarded development ....'. Common sense could predict this. Three-month-old or younger babies can spend up to ten hours a day in nursery. Even older children spend only seven or eight hours in school, with long holidays.

The psychoanalyst Jane Temperley has suggested that there may be unconscious motives besides the pressure to get more women into the workplace. 'The more that research shows the importance of the mother, the more there is an attempt to denigrate her role'. No-one, particularly a Conservative government, is likely to admit to envy of mothers and the maternal function. There is factual evidence of the effect of envy of the mother. A report in the Times of 17 February 2022 concluded that British women were four times more likely to die in childbirth than Scandinavian women; among European countries, only Slovakia has a higher rate of women's deaths in childbirth than Britain. Recently, a psychopathic nurse was able to conduct a killing spree in wards for vulnerable babies. Despite definitive evidence of who it might be, doctors were not allowed to prevent her and had to apologise to the murderer.

Not surprisingly, many nurseries make no attempt to replicate the important and helpful aspects of maternal care, although some staff must have had children of their own. The social work students were each asked to make ten weekly observations of one particular child. At first, students were anxious about how the small children would respond to an unknown adult. In reality, the children who were observed by these sympathetic social workers were delighted by the attention of a reliable adult. Sometimes a child gave the observer their favourite toy to hold. The students also had an opportunity to discuss their observations every week with an experienced seminar leader in small groups of six to eight members.

It was interesting that students rated nurseries higher if children were known as individuals with their own particular needs, for example, which children needed help in tying their shoelaces. This individual attention was in short supply. In some nurseries, staff seemed to have virtually given up on their difficult task. Nurses often congregated in the kitchen to talk to each other. Sick children might be left unattended, lying on the floor. Different children reacted differently to neglect. One little boy spent the whole time sitting silently under a table. However, he did speak to one member of staff who spoke his mother's language. We decided this was not the main issue, as he also spoke to the observer who only spoke English. It was focussed attention that seemed to meet his needs.

We felt it was important that students gained confidence in communicating with small children. Recently, there have been massive cuts in Health Visitor services that used to provide clinics with highly skilled nurses who made regular checks on small children. Without health visitors, the abuse of small children is less likely to be picked up. At the time of writing this, there have been two separate cases of small children who have been literally tortured to death despite being known to social services. In one, the baby daughter of one woman was being raised by the mother and her lesbian partner. Her uncle tried to raise the alarm, but the female social worker dismissed his concerns as 'homophobic'. Even if he was homophobic, this did not address the question of whether or not the little girl was being sadistically abused.

There has been a growing tendency in social work to fall back on political or sociological explanations. These issues can be important, but they cannot substitute for an understanding of the behaviour of individuals. In the past, social workers and health visitors could share their information. Health visitors administered the Edinburgh Post-Natal Depression scale and ran groups for mothers who needed post-natal support. Needless to say, Health visiting services have been cut to the bone. The cuts are not rational as early intervention can save time and the costs of intervention later. The cuts express yet another unconscious expression of the British envy of mothers.

At the end of the first term of our shared course, we asked students which aspects of the course were most useful for their work. To our surprise, a high proportion of our students said they found the young child observation particularly helpful. Many had little contact with children. They expected that children would be frightened of strange adults. Over time, students developed confidence in relating to the child they chose to focus on. The students' interest was often mirrored by the child having the experience of an adult who was focussed on them. Many nurseries offered a system of indiscriminate care. Any nurse could look after any child. In some nurseries, it took four different nurses to give a child its lunch. This is not the way small children are likely to experience lunch at home. It is depersonalising for staff and children. Different children reacted differently to this institutional neglect. One African-Caribbean boy sat at a table with little pieces of plasticene. He often smiled at staff. If they smiled back, he added another piece to the plasticene tower he was building. While some robust children can make the best of a bad job, many are adversely affected.

This is illustrated from the moment their mothers drop off their children. Many mothers separate from them very rapidly. This changed when the care improved. In 2010, two psychoanalytically trained consultants, Lynn Barnett and Isabel Menzies, made substantial changes to an already 'good' rated nursery. They put an end to the random care that children received. Each nurse was assigned their own little 'family' of three children whom they stayed with and followed through the day. The nurses were supported by the two consultants who were like helpful grandparents (Barnett, 2010).

One of the most surprising changes was in the behaviour of the mothers. Instead of rushing off, they lingered on and chatted to the staff and to each other. After a while, they set up their own mothers' support group. There were also changes about the way that staff felt. When one staff member was asked about how she felt about the changes, she said she could not explain it to her husband, but she felt it 'here', touching her heart. As these changes were so manifestly helpful, the consultants hoped they would trickle down to other nurseries. This was completely unrealistic. Staff would have needed opportunities for support and discussion. It might be more realistic and effective to introduce some of this straightforward understanding to nursery nurse training.

Improvement in the way small children were cared for also seemed to affect their mothers. This can be understood within a psychoanalytic framework. The psychoanalyst Melanie Klein described a method of wordless communication between a child and its mother. She called this 'Projective Identification'. If the child is unhappy about being left by the mother, this can be unconsciously picked up by the mother who often hurries away to escape her baby's distress. When the nursery was reorganised, the babies were no longer distressed at being left and the mothers stayed on.

To return to our course, when observations were finished, the students stayed in their groups of six to eight for the second and third terms with the same staff leader. They used these groups to discuss issues brought up by the lectures or from their work. In one group, they identified serious child abuse that had been missed in other places. These small groups met every week, so it was possible for the leaders and members to get to know each other. The students appreciated these regular groups. The importance of regular and reliable meetings for social work staff support and development is not always recognised. Even more sadly, this sort of support is rarely offered in homes for children in care where staff, often untrained, respond to children at random as in day nurseries without a theoretical framework to help them.

It is usually recognised that a child or teenager in their own family home needs contact with their mother. This need is often missed for the same children in care. After the Second World War, children having long treatments in hospitals were barely allowed to have any maternal contact. A married couple, the Robertsons realised that the most effective way to communicate children's distress at long separations from their parents, either in hospital or in residential nurseries, was to film them (Robertson, J and J, 1969).

We showed the students the Robertsons' film of a seventeen-month-old, John, in a residential nursery for nine days while his mother has a baby. The film makes distressing viewing. The care offered in the nursery is random. John's attempts to form a relationship with individual staff are continuously thwarted.

Even more relevant is the behaviour of the long-term resident children. They had formed a 'junior' gang (Rosenfeld, 2008). They held themselves together by shrieking, screaming, and laughing. Sometimes they attacked vulnerable children.

The purpose of the gang, whether in the mind or enacted externally, was described by psychoanalyst Herbert Rosenfeld who came to England as a refugee from nazi Germany in 1935. Rosenfeld (2008) describes how the gang state of mind is formed by someone mentally killing off their loving, dependent self. Instead, they identify with a destructive and narcissistic part of the self which provides them with a sense of superiority and self-admiration. This mental structure is delusional, but it can lure in the sane part of the self by offering freedom from emotional needs. This freedom makes the narcissistic gang state of mind compulsively addictive. Sexual exploitation often takes place as part of an external gang of men. A girl is passed from one man to another. Often, the originator 'grooms' the girl for this role. The psychoanalyst Dinora Pines (1993) has suggested that the vulnerability of girls that exploiters hook onto is not a leap into heterosexual sex. The girls are making an unconscious attempt to regain a physical relationship with their mother.

Pearce (2009) describes a conversation with a seventeen-year-old girl 'Lorna' whose mother has mental health problems. 'Sometimes I wish she was dead, but it's how I feel. But she's my Mum and I love her ....'. Her description of her relationship with her boyfriend reveals a similar ambivalence about him: '.... what he did to me really hurt .... In a way, I do forgive him because I love this boy deep down in my heart ....'. A girl with this sort of ambivalent relationship with her mother often finds it very difficult to look after a baby if she has one. This is probably due to her hostile or ambivalent relationship with her own mother as Pines suggests.

Pearce also describes a girl who is living at home with her baby and her mother. Social services withdraw, and within a few days, the girl and her mother have a row about feeding the baby. The girl runs away from home. It is possible that the girl's ambivalence to her own mother makes it impossible for her to allow her mother to support her. It is also impossible for the girl to think of how her baby might feel on being abruptly dropped by its mother. It is unrealistic to expect rapid change in people who have a long history of difficulties but the tendency for very brief social work is still common. This is often partly caused by staff limitations, but I think is also affected by the hopelessness projected by the client. In Pearce's view, it may take two years for a girl to recover from being exploited. Time is important, but it is also important for exploited girls to have an experience of a helpful maternal figure over a period of time. I describe later a situation where a social worker was aware of projections and had a helpful partnership with the client's health visitor and this led to improvement in the client's state of mind.

In the past, children's homes were usually large houses in the child's town or city. They were run by older women who were maternal figures. The location of the home made it possible for the child's social worker to visit regularly and for the child to stay in the same school. Now, care homes are often hundreds of miles from a child's home. There is little contact with their social worker or family. Staff are often untrained, and care can be random as seen in day nurseries. Gangs of exploiters may wait outside. They have a better picture of the girls' vulnerability than the local authorities.

We cannot go back to the past but ironically, we now know more about children's, parents' and workers' needs than we did then. This is vital as new groups of vulnerable children appear. A study by Nottingham University found that girls whose mothers and fathers worked long hours at interesting and demanding jobs were drawn into organised exploitation, for example, becoming 'gift girls' for county lines gangs (see Brewster et al., 2021).

There are a few things whose usefulness is proven. The use of psychoanalytic theory should be restored to social work training and nursery nurse training should be developed along the lines described by Barnet and Menzies. Numbers of health visitors should be restored to earlier levels – preventive work is more effective than cuts and cheaper in the long run.

A review into maternal deaths between 2019 and 2021 by Professor Marian Knight of Oxford University found that 241 women died either during pregnancy or within 6 weeks of giving birth. A further 331 died in the 12 months after giving birth. Suicide was the leading cause. The long-term effects on the child do not bear thinking about (Knight, 2023).

A true story

This was told to me by a colleague. It happened several years ago when there were more health visitors and they had time to work in partnership with social workers. A young woman, 'Mary', was referred to a newly qualified social worker. She had recently left Care. While in Care, she and some other girls had been targeted by a gang of sexual exploiters. Mary had recently had a baby but had no idea who the father was. She and the baby had been housed in a flat on a run-down estate. There were concerns about how she would manage. A Health Visitor had seen her and was encouraged that Mary had managed to give up drugs during her pregnancy. However, she seemed depressed.

The health visitor referred Mary to social services for ongoing support. Mary's case was assigned to a newly qualified social worker. As the social worker climbed the concrete stairs to the flat her heart sank. Mary was pale, her hair was unwashed. The baby was asleep. Its face seemed faintly blue. Mary slumped into a chair. The social worker sat on the only other chair. There were long silences in the conversation. Eventually, the social worker decided to go. However, she had formed a plan.

She told Mary that she would visit her every week on the same day and at the same time until Mary felt better. To her surprise, Mary got up and thanked her. She politely opened the door and said, 'See you next week'.

The social worker and health visitor talked. The health visitor would visit fortnightly and take clothes for the baby. On the social worker's next visit, Mary managed to smile at the social worker. The baby no longer looked blue. Her face was now a pale pink as if she had picked up some of her mother's warmer feelings.

After several months, the health visitor suggested that Mary could join a group for new mothers. At first, Mary refused to go. However, when the social worker told her she would carry on visiting until Mary felt settled, Mary agreed to give it a try.

None of this was a miracle cure. The social worker's heart sank every time she climbed the stairs. However, just as she persisted with her visits, Mary persisted with her baby and was able to try the more demanding setting of the support group. All the above may sound very simple but it is very demanding to visit a depressed person. The social worker had her training to help her. Most young people in the care system do not feel they can rely on their families. Unfortunately, the care system and most social workers usually offer only random contact. They don't have the training to develop a plan and the best they can offer at the end of a visit is 'See you soon'.

Some implications

At the time of writing this chapter, the Conservative government is making totally impractical attempts to get women with babies or very small children into the workforce. Presumably, the unconscious thinking behind this is that women who are able to leave their small children in nurseries and go back to work will want to vote for the Tories. Overtly the publicity seems to be suggesting that children will benefit from nurseries.

The evidence of this chapter and a great deal of research is that unless a child is not a baby but a resilient toddler, they may be adversely affected. Our observers found that babies can be appallingly neglected in nurseries. For example, one nurse was left looking after eight very small babies. Of course, there were regulations about this, but nurseries are not really to blame. Currently, nurseries are finding that staff are leaving in droves, and it is often difficult to recruit qualified staff. Although they may rightly complain that they can earn better pay elsewhere, I think this is rarely the reason. These situations existed long before the Covid pandemic which made a bad situation worse.

The current situation is at crisis point. The vague but elaborate 'improvements' suggested by the government do not seem linked to any meaningful research.

In this chapter, I have described the research by Isabel Menzies and Lynn Barnett (Barnett, 2010). They improved a nursery they consulted to by turning the care that was offered into something like the care a small child would receive from its mother. Instead of random indiscriminate care, each nurse had a small 'family' of three or four children that she did most things with. The apparently small change transformed the well-being of staff, children, and mothers. Our society creates an opposition of the needs of mothers and children which has even entered certain types of feminism. In the example above, it was the children's greater happiness that enabled mothers to stay and bond together.

It needs to be recognised that some of the ideas in this chapter are to offset the damage done by the attack on maternal care in our society. Reliability and emotional receptivity can easily be taught to nursery nurses and social workers, but they will need ongoing support in their work. The long-term benefits could be considerable.

Note

1 The NHS is the UK National Health Service

References

Barnett, L. (2010). *Isabel Menzies Lyth and action research*. British Journal of Psychotherapy 26(2): 146–151. DOI:10.1111/j.1752-0118.2010.01165.x

Brewster, B., Robinson, G., Silverman, B.W. and Walsh, D. (2021). *Covid-19 and child criminal exploitation in the UK: Implications of the pandemic for county lines*. Trends in Organized Crime 1–24. https://doi.org/10.1007/s12117-021-09442-x

Knight, M., Kathryn B., Allison F., Roshni P., Rohit K., Sara K., Jennifer K. (2023) *Report: Saving Lives, Improving Mothers' Care*. MMBRACE-UK, https://www.npeu.ox.ac.uk/assets/downloads/mbrrace-uk/reports/maternal-report-2023/MBRRACE-UK_Maternal_Compiled_Report_2023.pdf

McGuire J. and Earls F. (1994) *Evaluating a community intervention to reduce the risk of child abuse*. Child Abuse and Neglect 18: 473–485. https://doi.org/10.1016/0145-2134(94)90031-0

Pearce, J. (2009) *Young People and Sexual Exploitation*. London, Routledge.

Pines, D. (1993) *A Woman's Unconscious Use of Her Body*. London, Virago.

Robertson J. and J. (1969) *Film: John, Aged Seventeen Months, for Nine Days in a Residential Nursery*. http://www.robertsonfilms.info/

Rosenfeld, H. (2008) *Rosenfeld in Retrospect*. London, Routledge.

INDEX

Note: Page numbers followed by "n" refer to notes.

For Product Safety Concerns and Information please contact our EU
representative GPSR@taylorandfrancis.com Taylor & Francis Verlag GmbH,
Kaufingerstraße 24, 80331 München, Germany

Printed and bound by CPI Group (UK) Ltd, Croydon, CR0 4YY
08/06/2025
01897008-0006